MW00438927

Addictions Nursing

Scope and Standards of Practice

3rd Edition

Edited by Katherine S. Fornili, DNP, MPH, RN, CARN, FIAAN
and Susanne Fogger, DNP, PMHNP-BC, CARN-AP, FAANP

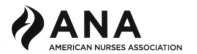

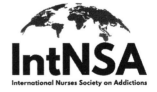

The American Nurses Association (ANA) and International Nurses Society on Addictions (IntNSA) are professional associations. This publication reflects the position of ANA and IntNSA regarding the scope and standards of addictions nursing practice and should be reviewed in conjunction with state board of nursing regulations. State law, rules, and regulations govern the practice of nursing, while *Addictions Nursing: Scope and Standards of Practice,* 3rd Edition guides registered nurses in the application of their professional skills and responsibilities.

About the American Nurses Association

The American Nurses Association (ANA) is the only full-service professional organization representing the interests of the nation's 4.3 million registered nurses through its constituent/state nurses associations and its organizational affiliates. The ANA advances the nursing profession by fostering high standards of nursing practice, promoting the rights of nurses in the workplace, projecting a positive and realistic view of nursing, and by lobbying the Congress and regulatory agencies on health care issues affecting nurses and the public.

American Nurses Association
8515 Georgia Avenue, Suite 400
Silver Spring, MD 20910

About the International Nurses Society on Addictions

The International Nurses Society on Addictions (IntNSA) is a professional specialty organization founded in 1975 for nurses committed to advancing excellence in addictions nursing practice through advocacy, collaboration, education, research, and policy development. IntNSA provides a forum for nurses who are interested in the prevention, intervention, and treatment of addictions and related disorders.

International Nurses Society on Addictions (IntNSA)
3416 Primm Lane
Birmingham, Alabama 35216

Cataloging in Publication data available from the Library of Congress

ISBNs
Print 978-1-947800-85-4
ePDF 978-1-947800-86-1
ePUB 978-1-947800-87-8
Mobi 978-1-947800-88-5
SAN: 851-3481

Contents

Code of Ethics and Addictions Nursing • 95

Standards of Addictions Nursing Practice • 103

Standards of Practice for Addictions Nursing • 107

Standards of Professional Performance for Addictions Nursing • 121

Contributors

EDITORS

Katherine S. Fornili, DNP, MPH, RN, CARN, FIAAN

Susanne Fogger, DNP, PMHNP-BC, CARN-AP, FAANP

CONTRIBUTORS

Oluremi Adejumo, DNP, MSc, BSN, RN

Carolyn Baird, DNP, MBA, RN-BC, CARN-AP, CCDPD, FIAAN

Charon Burda, DNP, PMHNP-BC, CRNP, CARN-AP

Carmel Clancy, PhD, RGN, RMN, BSc (Hons), PGCertHE, FPH, ICAPIII

Susanne Fogger, DNP, PMHNP-BC, CARN-AP, FAANP

Katherine S. Fornili, DNP, MPH, RN, CARN, FIAAN

Carolyn Jewell, MSN, RN, PMHNP-BC, CARN-AP

Khadijah Mahmoud, PhD, RN

Ann M. Mitchell, PhD, RN, FAAN

Dana Murphy-Parker, MS, PMHNP-BC, CARN-AP, FIAAN

Keith Plowden, PhD, PMHNP-BC, CARN-AP, CNE

Phyllis Raynor, PhD, PMHNP-BC, CARN-AP, APRN

Rosemary Smentkowski, RN, MSN, PMHNP-BC, CARN

Adam Searby, RN, BNurs (Hons), Grad Dip Ment H Nurs, Grad Dip AOD Studies, PhD

Victoria Selby, PhD, CRNP-PMH, PMHNP-BC, CARN-AP

Rachel Shuster, BSN, RN, CARN, CAAP

Stephen Strobbe, PhD, RN, PMHCNS-BC, CARN-AP, FIAAN, FAAN

Christine Vourakis, PhD, RN, FIAAN, FAAN

ANA COMMITTEE ON NURSING PRACTICE STANDARDS

Elizabeth "Liz" O. Dietz, EdD, RN, CS-NP, CSN (Co-Chair)

Mona Pearl Treyball, PhD, RN, CNS, CCRN-K, FAAN (Co-Chair)

Nena M. Bonuel, PhD, RN, APRN-BC, ACNS-BC, CCRN-K

Patricia Bowe, DNP, MS, RN

Danette Culver, MSN, RN, APRN, ACNS-BC, CCRN-K

Tonette "Toni" McAndrew, MPA, RN

Linda Inez Perkins, MSN, RN-BC

Michael Manasia, MSN, RN, OCN (Alternate)

Shelly Wells, PhD, MBA, APRN-CNS, ANEF (Alternate)

ANA STAFF

Carol J. Bickford, PhD, RN-BC, CPHIMS, FAMIA, FHIMSS, FAAN, Content Editor

Katie Boston-Leary, PhD, MBA, MHA, RN, NEA-BC, Contributor

Erin Walpole, BA, PMP, Production Editor

James Angelo, MA, Director of Publications

Introduction

SCOPE AND STANDARDS OF PRACTICE

The American Nurses Association's (ANA) *Nursing: Scope & Standards of Practice* is informed by advances in health care and professional nursing practice (ANA, 2021). It contains national standards of practice and performance that define the who, what, where, when, why, and how of nursing practice and is often used as a reference for the following:

- Quality improvement initiatives
- Certification and credentialing
- Position descriptions and performance appraisals
- Classroom teaching and in-service education programs
- Boards of nursing members' orientation programs and regulatory decision-making activities

Specialty nursing scope and standards of practice documents provide comprehensive overviews of the dynamic and complex practice of various nursing specialties. *Addictions Nursing: Scope and Standards of Practice* is one of several specialty nursing scope and standards of practice documents. It is jointly published by ANA and the International Nurses Society on Addictions (IntNSA). While IntNSA is an international nursing specialty organization, this document is intended primarily as a reference source for American nurses. However, it may contain valuable information for nurses in other countries. *Addictions Nursing: Scope and Standards of Practice* is intended to guide nurses who serve individuals and families affected by substance use and related behaviors, as well as administrators, legislators, regulators, legal counsel, and other interprofessional colleagues. ANA and IntNSA (www.IntNSA.org) partner to jointly produce this document approximately every 5 years to describe a competent level of nursing care at each level of addictions nursing practice.

WHAT IS ADDICTION?

At the time of this writing, there is no established nursing definition for "addiction." In 2011, the American Society of Addiction Medicine (ASAM) defined *addiction* as "a primary, chronic disease of brain reward, motivation, memory and related circuitry" (ASAM, 2011, p. 1). Over time, public understanding and acceptance of addiction as a chronic brain disease allowed an enhanced focus on remission, recovery, and wellness, as well as the roles of prevention and harm reduction in the spectrum of addiction and recovery (ASAM, 2019, p. 2). In response to these evolving concepts, ASAM established a Descriptive and Diagnostic Terminology Action Group (DDTAG) to update definitions for terms related to treatment, recovery, and the full spectrum of unhealthy substance use. The ASAM Board of Directors adopted a new definition of addiction in 2019:

> Addiction is a treatable, chronic medical disease involving complex interactions among brain circuits, genetics, the environment, and an individual's life experiences. People with addiction use substances or engage in behaviors that become compulsive and often continue despite harmful consequences. (ASAM, 2019, p. 2)

WHAT ARE SUBSTANCE USE DISORDERS?

The fifth edition of the *Diagnostic and Statistical Manual of Mental Disorders* (*DSM-5*; American Psychiatric Association [APA], 2013) is commonly used among all providers in various disciplines in the United States. The *DSM-5* refers to "substance use disorders" (SUD), rather than "addiction," "substance abuse," or "dependence" to describe significant clinical and functional impairment resulting from the recurrent use of substances. Substance use disorders are defined as mild, moderate, or severe, based on the number of *DSM-5* diagnostic criteria met by an individual. The SUD diagnosis is not based solely on pharmacological criteria (e.g., tolerance, withdrawal, toxicity); rather, the diagnosis is established when the patient demonstrates evidence of impaired control, social impairment, and risky use.

WHAT ARE BEHAVIORAL ADDICTIONS?

"Addiction" is characterized as a complex condition with the following four defining characteristics:

- Continued engagement in behavior despite adverse consequences;
- Diminished self-control over engagement in the behavior;
- Compulsive engagement in the behavior; and
- An appetitive urge or craving state prior to engagement in the behavior (Yau et al., 2020).

Addiction has been commonly associated with the use of substances, but the term has more recently been used to describe excessive engagement in problematic nondrug behaviors (gambling, sex, eating, internet use). The *DSM-5* renamed its "substance-related disorders" diagnostic category as the "substance-related and addictive disorders" category (Yau et al., 2020). However, currently, only gambling disorder (formerly called "pathologic gambling") is included in the *DSM-5* in the section called "non-substance-related disorders" (APA, 2013). Addictive behavioral disorders share certain characteristics with substance use disorders (impulsivity, loss of control, self-destructive behaviors), have similar biological and environmental etiologies, and often co-occur in relation to use of alcohol or drugs (Fouladi et al., 2015). For these reasons, in the United States, caring for individuals with compulsive, disordered behaviors falls within the purview of the addictions nurse.

WHAT IS RECOVERY?

In August 2010, leaders in the behavioral health field, consisting of people in recovery from mental health and substance use disorders and representatives from the U.S. Department of Health and Human Services (DHHS) Substance Abuse and Mental Health Services Administration (SAMHSA), met to explore the development of a common, unified working definition of recovery. Prior to this, SAMHSA, as well as other government agencies, had separate definitions for recovery from mental disorders and substance use disorders. Lack of a common language about recovery complicated discussions about treatment and recovery support services, as well as efforts to expand health insurance coverage for these disorders (SAMHSA, 2012a).

According to SAMHSA, *recovery* is "a process of change through which people improve their health and wellness, live self-directed lives, and strive to reach their full potential" (SAMHSA, 2020c, para. 1). There are four major dimensions of wellness that support recovery:

- **Health**—overcoming or managing one's disease(s) or symptoms and making informed, healthy choices that support physical and emotional well-being;
- **Home**—having a stable and safe place to live;
- **Purpose**—conducting meaningful daily activities and having the independence, income, and resources to participate in society; and
- **Community**—having relationships and social networks that provide support, friendship, love, and hope (SAMHSA, 2020c).

The foundation of recovery is hope, or the belief that addiction and its related challenges and conditions can be managed effectively. Recovery is highly personal; it occurs via many pathways, and it is supported through social networks and relationships. Recovery is characterized by continual growth and improvement in health and wellness, although the process of recovery can involve multiple setbacks, making resilience a key component of recovery (SAMHSA, 2020c). The first director-general of the World Health Organization (WHO) famously stated that "without mental health there can be no true physical health" (Chisholm, 1951). According to SAMHSA, "behavioral health is essential to health, prevention works, treatment is effective, and people recover from mental and/or substance use disorders" (SAMHSA, 2020c). Nurses across the United States and around the world have the capacity and obligation to promote recovery and positively influence outcomes related to substance use and addictive disorders.

WHAT IS ADDICTIONS NURSING?

As a global society, IntNSA has adopted modified versions of the International Council of Nurses' (ICN) definitions of "nurse" and "nursing" to avoid limiting membership in the Society only to nurses in the United States. IntNSA defines a "nurse" as a person who has completed a program of basic, generalized nursing education and is authorized by the appropriate regulatory authority to practice nursing in their country.

The ICN definition of "nursing" states,

> Nursing encompasses autonomous and collaborative care of individuals of all ages, families, groups, and communities, sick or well and in all settings. Nursing includes the promotion of health, prevention of illness, and the care of ill, disabled and dying people. Advocacy, promotion of a safe environment, research, participation in shaping health policy and in patient and health systems management, and education are also key nursing roles. (ICN, 2002)

IntNSA defines "addictions nursing" as a distinct nursing specialty practice which incorporates nursing science and the therapeutic use of self with knowledge about substance use and addictive disorders. An addictions nurse is a "nurse" as defined previously who also has the expertise to provide care across the continuum of addictive disorders, by focusing their efforts on preventing substance use or problematic behaviors, intervening with those who already have risks for developing an addictive disorder, and providing treatment and recovery support services when indicated. Addictions nurses provide care for individuals with substance use, as well as those with other compulsive and harmful behaviors (e.g., "process addictions" like eating or sexual disorders and problematic internet use or gambling). The addictions nurse's person-centered approach supports comprehensive care for individuals and families across the life span. Addictions nurses are instrumental in translating evidence-based knowledge to practice, including disseminating that knowledge to nurses in other specialties and interprofessional colleagues.

Historically, addictions nursing was practiced almost exclusively in specialized alcohol and drug treatment facilities, with patients in more advanced stages of illness. However, IntNSA recognizes that all nurses in a variety of healthcare settings increasingly encounter patients with, or at risk of, addictive disorders on a daily basis. Addictions nursing practice is "knowledge specific," not "setting specific" (Vourakis, 1996). Nurses in all practice settings acknowledge the need for more education about the care of individuals and populations with substance use and addictive disorders. IntNSA recognizes that *all* nurses need to have requisite knowledge and competencies in addictions and encourages nurses in *any* specialty to consider obtaining specialty certification in addictions.

The Institute of Medicine (IOM) report *The Future of Nursing: Leading Change, Advancing Health* (2011) was a catalyst for the advancement of the nursing profession and patient-centered care. *The Future of Nursing 2020–2030: Charting a Path to Achieve Health Equity* focuses on creating a culture of health, reducing health disparities, and improving the health and well-being of the U.S. population in the 21st century (National Academies of Sciences, Engineering, and Medicine, 2021). Nurses specializing in addictions lead change in the delivery of health care for individuals, families, communities, and populations affected by problematic substance use and addictive behaviors, which will reduce disparities and improve health equity. Addictions nurses have an essential role in population health, through early intervention efforts such as screening, brief intervention, and referral to treatment (SBIRT). Addictions nurses also intervene at the population level by promoting access to care and advocating for policies and programs that can reduce substance-related harm, particularly for populations experiencing health inequities.

Nursing education may have not kept pace with trends to reframe substance use and its adverse consequences within the context of a growing public health crisis. Nursing curricula often lack standardized addictions content, and programs offer only a minimal number of clinical hours allotted to addictions in prelicensure and graduate nursing programs.

Thus, nurses often lack the knowledge needed to understand the complexity of substance use and addictive disorders (Campbell-Heider et al., 2009; Finnell et al., 2018; Mollica et al., 2011; Poznyak et al., 2019; Savage et al., 2014). Therefore, nurses wishing to specialize in addictions nursing must find alternative methods to increase their knowledge and clinical competencies about substance use and related adverse health effects, including the biological, psychosocial, behavioral, and public health aspects of these disorders.

The International Nurses Society on Addictions

The sections that follow describe the history of the International Nurses Society on Addictions (IntNSA), its affiliations, and other resources.

HISTORY OF INTNSA

IntNSA has a long and rich history that stretches back to 1974, when the American Nurses Association (ANA) supported the establishment of the National Nurses Society on Alcoholism (NNSA) during its biennial conference. In 1975, NNSA was officially formed as the nursing counterpart to a physician's group called the American Medical Society on Alcoholism.

In 1983, NNSA changed its name to the National Nurses Society on Addictions, which reflected all substances and behaviors that can lead to addiction yet allowed the Society to maintain its "NNSA brand." Efforts to support and increase awareness about addictions and the role and value of nursing resulted in the first publication of the *Standards of Practice in Addictions Nursing* (1984). In 1987, ANA, NNSA, and the Drug and Alcohol Nurses Association (DANA, not to be confused with the Drug and Alcohol Nurses of Australasia) collaboratively produced a publication called *The Care of Clients with Addictions: Dimensions of Nursing Practice*.

By 1990, NNSA had developed the Certified Addictions Registered Nurse (CARN) credential; launched a new periodical, *Perspectives on Addictions Nursing*; and recruited approximately 1,000 nurses into its membership. Around 1997, NNSA members began taking an interest in what addictions nurses in other organizations and in other countries were doing.

In 2000, to consolidate efforts, and to avoid name confusion, the three addictions nursing groups in the United States (NNSA, the Consolidated Association of Nurses in Substance Abuse [CANSA], and DANA) merged, acknowledged the efforts of addictions nurses in other countries, and named the new organization the International Nurses Society on Addictions (IntNSA).

INTNSA'S VISION AND MISSION

With a stated vision of becoming a "global leader in addictions nursing," and recognizing the potential for wider international impact, the newly formed IntNSA organization created an "international task force" and began to recruit more nurses from outside the United States and Canada.

INTNSA'S VISION AND MISSION

IntNSA's vision is to be a global leader in addictions nursing. The mission of the society shall be to advance excellence in addictions nursing practice through advocacy, collaboration, education, research, and policy development. It shall serve as a forum for nurses who are interested in the prevention, intervention, and treatment of addiction so that they may enhance their knowledge, advance their skills, continue their education, and be a resource to nurses in all areas of practice.

In 2010, IntNSA's Learning From Each Other: A Global Perspective of Addictions conference provided a springboard for strengthening and growing international networks. IntNSA partnered with addictions nurses in the United Kingdom (e.g., the Association of Nurses in Substance Abuse [ANSA]) and elsewhere (e.g., the Drug and Alcohol Practitioners' Association of Aoteroa, New Zealand [DAPAANZ]; Drug and Alcohol Nurses of Australasia [also called DANA]) to form a small global community forum for sharing information relevant to addictions nurses worldwide, and the Global Addictions Nursing Network (GANN) on Facebook was launched. GANN is a non-organizationally aligned international global network for addictions nurses and those interested in addictions (http://www.facebook.com/GlobalAddictionNursingNetwork).

In 2014, members elected its first international member to the IntNSA board of directors. In March 2015, a strategy and model for international development was presented at the IntNSA strategic planning retreat held by the board of directors. The full board enthusiastically adopted this plan and presented it to the wider membership at the next annual business meeting, and the international strategy took on new energy to drive through these changes. In 2019, IntNSA's board reviewed its progress, updated its plan, and developed consensus for its ongoing development.

INTNSA'S GLOBAL STRUCTURE

As an international nursing society, IntNSA recognizes that drug and alcohol problems (as well as other behavioral disorders) and the political, economic, social, and medical responses to these problems vary from country to country and region to region (Clancy & Fornili, 2019). Therefore, IntNSA has conceptually mapped its membership model to the World Health Organization's (WHO's) six regional groups: (1) African Region, (2) Region of the Americas, (3) South-East Asia Region, (4) European Region, (5) Eastern Mediterranean Region, and (6) Western Pacific Region. IntNSA has over 750 members in at least 16 countries representing the six WHO Regions, including Africa (Nigeria, South Africa, and Tanzania), the Americas (Antigua, Brazil, Canada, Chile, and the United States), Eastern Mediterranean (Qatar), Europe (Iceland, Ireland, Israel, Netherlands, Portugal, and the United Kingdom), South-East Asia (Thailand), and the Western-Pacific (Japan and South Korea).

IntNSA's first international region was the Americas (Brazil, Canada, and the United States), followed by the European Region, which was launched at the 2018 International Council of Nurses (ICN) Advanced Nursing Practice Conference in Rotterdam. Next, in 2019, Nigeria and Tanzania became the first two IntNSA chapters in the African Region. At the time of this writing, IntNSA has nine "national chapters" (Brazil, Canada, Ireland, the Netherlands, Nigeria, Portugal, Tanzania, and the United Kingdom), including the IntNSA United States of America (IntNSA USA) chapter. In 2019, IntNSA entered into a memorandum of agreement to create an organizational affiliate status relationship (as opposed to a "chapter") with DANA, which represents Australia, New Zealand, and the Western Pacific Islands. Additionally, there are several "state chapters" in the IntNSA USA Chapter.

JOURNAL OF ADDICTIONS NURSING: OFFICIAL JOURNAL OF THE INTERNATIONAL NURSES SOCIETY ON ADDICTIONS

The *Journal of Addictions Nursing* (*JAN*) is the official journal of IntNSA. It is published quarterly to keep members apprised of best practice in addictions nursing. The journal disseminates current research, official position papers, and articles pertinent to clinical practice and current trends and innovations. Regular columns keep readers abreast of emerging clinical issues (Clinical Reviews); scientific studies (Research Reviews); legislative concerns (Policy Watch); pharmacological interventions (Pharmacology Corner); nurse support programs (Peer Assistance); and online resources and social media (Media Watch). Additionally, the journal publishes columns about leaders in the field (Innovative Roles) and personal viewpoints (Stories from the Field).

Theme-based special issues of the journal are published intermittently to focus attention on important topics, such as recovery and recovery-oriented systems of care, women with co-occurring disorders, tobacco use, opioid use disorders, and social determinants of addiction.

The editor-in-chief of the journal is responsible and accountable to IntNSA and serves as an ex officio member of IntNSA's governing body, the board of directors.

INTERNATIONAL ACADEMY OF ADDICTIONS NURSING

The International Academy of Addictions Nursing (IAAN) was formed in 2014 to foster excellence in nursing practice, administration, research, and education in addictions nursing. The Academy recognizes the wisdom of outstanding individuals in the profession who have contributed in sustained and significant ways. Individuals are inducted into the Academy as fellows based on their outstanding contributions to addictions nursing and are entitled to use the credential FIAAN. Applicants for fellowship in the Academy provide documented evidence of their enduring and substantial contributions in one or more of the following areas:

- Teaching and learning innovation in addictions nursing
- Faculty development in addictions nursing
- Primary research in addictions nursing
- Translational research in addictions nursing
- Leadership in addictions nursing
- Public policy related to addictions nursing at a local, state, or national level
- Collaborative education/practice/administration/research/ community partnerships
- Exemplary practice as an addictions nurse

Applicants for fellowship in IAAN must be current IntNSA members. Current certification as a CARN (Certified Addictions Registered Nurse) or a CARN-AP (Certified Addictions Registered Nurse-Advanced Practice) is ideal but not required. Applicants must provide evidence of how they will continue to provide visionary leadership in addictions nursing and how their contributions are congruent with the mission and goals of IntNSA.

The president of IAAN is responsible and accountable to IntNSA and serves as an ex officio member of IntNSA's governing body, the board of directors.

FOUNDATION FOR ADDICTIONS NURSING

The Foundation for Addictions Nursing (FAN) is a nonprofit entity that is financially independent of IntNSA. It serves to support the mission of IntNSA through philanthropic development and altruistic support. Its primary role is to cultivate resources and utilize assets provided by donors to help IntNSA advance the profession of addictions nursing. The Foundation cultivates relationships with individuals and organizations and manages assets provided by donors. It supports the development of emerging addictions nursing researchers, early career educators, and clinicians in pursuit of clinical excellence. It supports pilot research grants for addictions nursing research and provides conference scholarships to assist students in professional development.

The president of the Foundation collaborates with and serves as an ex officio member of IntNSA's governing body, the board of directors.

INTNSA'S ORGANIZATIONAL AFFILIATIONS

American Nurses Association

Founded in 1896, ANA represents over 4.2 million registered nurses in all 50 states and U.S. territories (ANA, n.d.-a). ANA exists to advance the nursing profession by fostering high standards of nursing practice; promoting a safe and ethical work environment; bolstering the health and wellness of nurses; and advocating on healthcare issues that affect nurses and the public (ANA, n.d.-a).

As a nursing specialty organization, IntNSA USA is an organizational affiliate (OA) of ANA. Serving as an organizational-level member within ANA allows IntNSA USA to maintain its autonomy as a specialty nursing organization while holding a voting seat in ANA's annual Membership Assembly.

This relationship with ANA provides IntNSA USA with a platform for speaking on behalf of healthcare issues and opportunities to collaborate in order to improve quality and find solutions for the addictions nursing specialty. Thus, addictions nurses and the patients we serve benefit from the "shared voice" of ANA, one of the largest professional nursing organizations in the world.

International Council of Nurses

Founded in 1899, the International Council of Nurses (ICN) is a federation of more than 130 national nurses associations, including ANA. ICN represents more than 20 million nurses worldwide and is the world's widest reaching international organization for health professionals. Operated by leading nurses internationally, ICN works to ensure quality nursing care for all. ICN guides and represents nurses around the world by promoting sound health policies and the advancement of nursing knowledge, and by demonstrating the worldwide impact of this respected profession.

In 2019, IntNSA became a specialist affiliate of ICN. This offers IntNSA expanded opportunities for collaboration with nurses from all over the world and with other organizations on the international stage, such as WHO and the United Nations. Importantly, specialty affiliation status with ICN helps IntNSA to fulfill its vision of being "a global leader in addictions nursing." As it continues to grow internationally, IntNSA will belong to or partner with other nursing specialty organizations in other regions around the globe.

European Specialist Nurses Organisation

The European Specialist Nurses Organisation (ESNO) is a nonprofit organization that represents the interests of specialist nurses in the European Union (EU) and greater Europe. As part of IntNSA's launch of the European Region in 2018, ESNO formally invited IntNSA to become a member of its network. ESNO provides a framework for communication and cooperation between European specialist nursing organizations and enables the political voice of specialist nurses, including addictions nurses.

Addictions Nursing Certification Board

As an addictions nursing specialty organization, IntNSA promotes excellence in addictions nursing practice through its relationship with the Addictions Nursing Certification Board (ANCB). ANCB currently certifies nurses in the United States and Canada. The primary purpose of ANCB is to provide a mechanism and framework for certification and recertification of the addictions nursing specialty. Certification helps to ensure that nurses have attained certain levels of nursing competence and are capable of evidence-based addictions nursing practice. Certification serves to promote and maintain quality nursing care by providing a mechanism for nurses to demonstrate their proficiency as addictions nurses. Nurses who meet certification criteria demonstrate attainment of specialized knowledge beyond the basic nursing credential.

Historically, ANCB operated as a committee under the IntNSA bylaws. In December 1989, ANCB established and administered the first addictions nursing certification examinations for nurses to receive the CARN credential.

As the advanced practice nursing workforce expanded, IntNSA and ANCB identified a need for an advanced practice credential. In 2000, ANCB created the CARN-Advanced Practice (CARN-AP). The number of nurses holding the CARN or the CARN-AP certification continues to grow steadily. Nurses in all specialty areas who meet ANCB criteria for certification are eligible to become CARNs or CARN-APs.

ANCB supports IntNSA's mission by providing a mechanism for nurses in the US and Canada to demonstrate competencies in addictions nursing. It became autonomous from IntNSA in 2014, due to accreditation standards that require that the certifying organization be an autonomous entity. Subsequently, the Accreditation Board for Specialty Nursing Certification (ABSNC) granted accreditation for the CARN and the CARN-AP in 2018. ABSNC, an independent authority of accreditation of nursing certification programs, confers quality, rigor, and a mark of excellence.

Scope of Practice: Addictions Nursing

The role of the addictions nurse has become increasingly complex and varied. Recent literature has focused on *substance use* or *substance-specific functions* (i.e., assessment, screening, treatment monitoring, and addictions counseling), without describing a nursing-specific role. While numerous nursing theorists have described the role of nurses in general, there are few studies that focus specifically on the role of the addictions nurse. One of the first studies published about the role of the addictions nurse was a qualitative study in the United Kingdom, which identified five distinct, sequential stages of role development for addictions nurse specialists (Clancy et al., 2007). Each stage is characterized by key features of role acquisition, with the early stages being pivotal to retention. The five stages include: encounter, engagement, stabilization, competency, and mastery. First, the nurse enters the field with a general lack of knowledge or skills related to addictions and then develops confidence and credibility. Once staff and patients acknowledge that the addictions nurse is credible and clinically competent, the nurse begins to mentor others. Finally, the addictions nurse is viewed as having mastery and may begin to serve in a consultant role. Failure to navigate the early stages of role development is associated with early departure from addictions nursing. Thus, it is recommended that student nurses and nurses new to the specialty obtain professional development opportunities and clinical experiences that are matched to these stage-specific competencies.

Regardless of professional specialty, all nurses, in fact, all healthcare professionals, must have a basic understanding of addictive disorders, including knowledge of current models, theories, and treatment modalities; appreciation of multiple contexts within which substance use and related disorders occur; awareness of the effects of psychoactive drug use and addictive behaviors; and how these result in enduring neurobiological, cognitive, and behavioral changes. There remains a need for a specialist in addictions nursing at the level of the registered nurse, the graduate or master's, the advanced practice registered nurse (APRN), and the doctorally prepared nurse (Marcus et al., 2020). In the United States, treatment programs frequently hire licensed professional nurses/licensed vocational nurses (LPN/LVN). Therefore, IntNSA acknowledges the need to expand addictions nursing education to these nurses, as well as nurses in other countries who are not regulated by U.S. nursing licensure requirements.

LEVELS OF ADDICTIONS NURSING

Note: This section describes the scope of practice within the United States for nurses with various levels of academic preparation. See also the Standards of Addictions Nursing Practice section for specific competencies for each level of preparation.

Addictions Registered Nurse

Entry into addictions nursing practice requires, at a minimum, completion of an accredited prelicensure nursing program and successful attainment of all licensure requirements. Half of all newly licensed registered nurses (RNs) in the United States enter the workforce with a diploma or an associate degree (Smiley et al., 2019), yet it is the position of the American Association of Colleges of Nursing (AACN) that the minimum level of preparation for RNs should be at the baccalaureate level (e.g., the bachelor of science in nursing [BSN] or an equivalent baccalaureate degree in nursing), offered at an accredited four-year college or university (AACN, 2019). According to AACN and the Institute of Medicine (IOM, 2011), staffing levels that rely on baccalaureate-prepared nurses are associated with lower mortality rates, fewer medication errors, and improved patient outcomes. Further, healthcare systems that are population-focused and that utilize community-based approaches to care rely on RNs who can practice across multiple settings and function to the fullest extent of their license (AACN, 2019; IOM, 2011). It is important that nurses engage in lifelong learning to prepare themselves to meet these expectations.

Many acute and chronic health and social conditions are associated with problematic substance use and other compulsive disorders (e.g., gambling, eating, gaming, and sex disorders). Nurses across all specialties routinely encounter persons experiencing consequences from these conditions. It is important that all nurses recognize substance use and symptoms of substance use disorder (SUD) and other compulsive conditions. It is also important that nurses are able to recognize risk for adverse consequences that may result from a single episode of risky substance use, such as a motor vehicle crash, drowning, or poisoning. All nurses and other healthcare providers should be knowledgeable and competent to intervene across the continuum of substance use and across the lifespan in order to meet *Healthy People 2030* objectives. These include reducing substance use and substance-related consequences and improving access to specialty treatment for substance use problems (Office of Disease Prevention and Health Promotion, 2019).

Graduate-Level Prepared Addictions Nurse

Graduate-level education prepares nurses to focus on the complex needs of individuals, groups, and communities. Graduate-level prepared nurses may also obtain advanced degrees in other areas, such as public health, business, and administration. For example, public health nurses focus on enhancing the health of populations. The population-based approach of public health nursing is ideal for addressing the holistic impact of substance use and the consequences of SUDs. Graduate-level prepared nurses are skilled in inpatient care and communication technologies to integrate and coordinate care, and they collaborate and intervene at the system level for policy development, advocacy, and interprofessional collaboration to improve the health of patients, populations, and systems (AACN, 2011, 2021).

Graduate-level prepared nurses apply research outcomes within the practice setting, resolve practice problems, and disseminate results. They are prepared to work with special populations across the lifespan (e.g., women's health, prenatal, neonatal, pediatric, older adults). They deliver care in diverse settings that provide services for vulnerable populations (e.g., psychiatric, HIV, trauma, corrections). Graduate-level prepared nurses in roles as nurse educators have significant opportunities to close the aforementioned gap in nursing education related to individuals, families, and communities affected by substance use and SUDs. Graduate-level prepared nurses in leadership positions can be instrumental in the design and implementation of prevention, intervention, treatment, and recovery programs. These nurse leaders are in key roles to promote the wide dissemination of evidence-based practices.

Graduate level prepared nurses in addictions nursing may include those with preparation at the master's, advanced practice, or doctoral levels, described next.

MASTER'S LEVEL ADDICTIONS NURSE

Master's level nursing education is a critical component of the nursing education continuum (AACN, 2011). This may include a master's in nursing science (MSN), a master's in science with a nursing focus (MS), or a Clinical Nurse Leader (CNL). Graduates of master's degree programs in nursing are prepared with broad knowledge and practice expertise that build and expand on baccalaureate or entry-level nursing practice and meet the competencies outlined in the AACN *Essentials: Core Competencies for Professional Nursing Education* (2021). The AACN *Advanced-Level Nursing Education Competencies* guide all graduate nursing programs, provide necessary curricular elements and frameworks, delineate outcomes expected of graduates, and set expectations for preparing advanced nursing graduates for diverse areas of practice in any healthcare setting, including specialty practice settings (AACN, 2021).

The master's prepared addictions nurse uses the AACN *Advanced-Level Nursing Education Competencies* as a foundation for practice and integrates scientific findings from nursing, biopsychosocial fields, genetics, public health, quality improvement, and organizational sciences for the continual improvement. The AACN *Advanced-Level Nursing Education Competencies* outlines organizational and systems leadership skills critical to the promotion of high quality and safe patient care and emphasizes ethical and critical decision-making, effective working relationships, and a systems perspective. Graduate nurses who incorporate the AACN *Advanced-Level Nursing Education Competencies* into their practice are change agents and apply quality principles within their organizations (AACN, 2021).

ADVANCED PRACTICE REGISTERED NURSE

The advanced practice registered nurse (APRN) holds at least a master's degree in addition to the initial nursing education and licensing required for all RNs. The APRN is a regulatory title that includes the following four roles: certified registered nurse anesthetist (CRNA), certified nurse midwife (CNM), clinical nurse specialist (CNS), and certified nurse practitioner (CNP). All four of these APRN roles share a focus on direct care to individual healthcare consumers. CRNAs provide a full range of anesthesia and pain management services. CNMs provide primary, gynecological, and reproductive health care. CNSs provide diagnosis, treatment, and ongoing management of patients and expertise and support to nurses caring for patients. CNPs provide primary, acute, and specialty health care across the lifespan through assessment, diagnosis, and treatment of illnesses and injuries. Advanced practice nurses help drive practice changes throughout the organization and ensure use of evidence-based care to achieve the best possible patient outcomes (American Nurses Association [ANA], n.d.-b).

State laws and regulations define criteria for licensure for each designated APRN role. *Consensus Model for APRN Regulation: Licensure, Accreditation, Certification, and Education* ensures healthcare consumer safety and access to APRNs (APRN Consensus Workgroup & NCSBN APRN Advisory Committee, 2008). In addition to the licensure, accreditation, certification, and education (LACE) requirements for APRNs outlined in *Consensus Model*, other professional, accreditation, and certification organizations outline standards and competencies for the advanced practice role. *Addictions Nursing: Scope and Standards of Practice*, published jointly by ANA and IntNSA, promotes standards and competencies for the advanced practice addictions registered nurse role. The Addiction Nursing Certification Board (ANCB) addresses standards and competencies for the Certified Addictions Registered Nurse—Advanced Practice (CARN-AP) credential.

APRNs who specialize in addictions serve as leaders, consultants, change agents, and direct care providers—critical roles for reducing the societal harm related to use of alcohol, tobacco, and other drugs. They build on their foundational graduate nursing education for their role through advanced knowledge and competence, gained through specialty continuing education, formal courses in higher education, or both. The APRN working with patients with addictive disorders must be able to translate new evidence into practice as innovations in prevention, treatment, and recovery management develop (Nagel & Fougere, 2017).

All APRNs have opportunities to assess, identify, and treat substance use issues within their patient populations. For example, if available, nurse midwives may choose to refer pregnant patients to a specialty clinic for treatment and monitoring, but if such resources are not available, they can become prepared and waivered to prescribe buprenorphine to their patients. However, it is recommended that APRNs who may choose to provide medication-assisted treatment (MAT; e.g., buprenorphine for opioid use disorders) check their state's scope of practice regulations and obtain additional education beyond the minimal educational requirements mandated under the Comprehensive Addiction and Recovery Act (CARA).

DOCTORALLY PREPARED NURSE

Education is the path for nurses to achieve greater levels of expertise. The nursing profession needs more nurses educated at the doctoral level to replenish the supply of faculty, researchers, and advanced practice clinicians. Doctorally prepared nurses build upon the foundation acquired through a baccalaureate or master's degree in nursing, steward the profession, educate the next generation of nurses, define the profession's uniqueness, and maintain its professional integrity (AACN, 2006):

- *Doctor of Philosophy:* Research-focused nurses with the doctor of philosophy degree (PhD) or a doctor of nursing science degree (DNS, DSN, or DNSc) are needed to further develop the science of nursing to improve health care (AACN, 2006). Doctorally prepared, research-focused nurses are prepared at the highest level to conduct research that advances the science of nursing. They support health sciences research by demonstrating high levels of expertise congruent with their scholarly focus and providing leadership to sustain funding (AACN, 2010).

- *Doctor of Nursing Practice:* Practice-focused nurses with the doctor of nursing practice (DNP) degree are prepared for advanced practice roles and leadership in clinical and academic settings. The DNP applies theoretical, conceptual, and operational perspectives relative to implementation science as a basis for the design and management of evidence-based practice (EBP) change (Riner, 2015). The DNP implements the seven steps of EBP to improve healthcare quality, safety, and patient outcomes; reduce costs; and increase nurse satisfaction. This approach is based on cultivating a spirit of inquiry and involves searching for the best research evidence, critically appraising that evidence, integrating evidence with clinical expertise and patient preferences and values, evaluating outcomes of practice change, and disseminating EBP results (Melnyk et al., 2010).

Research- and practice-focused doctorally prepared nurses have key roles in addictions nursing and are essential in redesigning health care to close the quality gap for individuals affected by addictive disorders. They advance an understanding of evidence-based behavioral health care, improve outcomes, and promote the well-being of patients, families, and communities.

Doctorally prepared nurse educators have significant opportunities to advance the professional practice of the current and future nursing workforce by enhancing addictions nursing curricular content in schools of nursing and continuing education programs and by promoting meaningful clinical experiences (Campbell-Heider et al., 2009; Finnell et al., 2018; Mollica et al., 2011; Savage et al., 2011).

EVIDENCE-BASED PRACTICE OF ADDICTIONS NURSING

There are many definitions of evidence-based practice (EBP), which is an umbrella term that covers evidence-based medicine, nursing, public health, dentistry, and so on. From a nursing perspective, Melnyk et al.

(2010) define EBP as "a problem-solving approach to the delivery of health care that integrates best evidence from studies and patient care data with clinician expertise and patient preferences and values" (p. 51). It is a healthcare approach that assesses and combines scientific evidence from research studies, best patient care practices, clinician expertise, and patients' individualized choices and beliefs into the decision-making process in order to improve patients' care (Farokhzadian et al., 2015; Koivunen et al., 2010). Ethical consideration, skill, competency, sound clinical judgment, and the ability to develop a therapeutic alliance are also critical components of EBP.

When healthcare interventions focus on these dimensions and are implemented, the goal of safe, effective, and efficient treatment can attain the best patient outcomes. According to Melnyk and Fineout-Overholt (2005), EBP also includes what Aristotle defined as *techne* (the skills and expertise required to produce intended outcomes) and *phronesis* (the ability to modify one's course of action based on an evaluation of change in the patient's current status, abilities, preferences, and values). In other words, it is critical to use good clinical judgment and careful discernment of human concerns at stake when implementing standardized guidelines, even those with adequate evidence. Addictions nurses must continuously self-evaluate their knowledge and competencies, stay current on the latest research required for the provision of quality patient care, and optimize their clinical decision-making.

There are many EBP guidelines and recommendations currently being utilized, including screening, brief intervention, and referral to treatment (SBIRT); medications for the treatment of SUD; standardized assessment tools for withdrawal for infants and adults; and motivational interviewing (MI) techniques for intervening with patients. The Substance Abuse and Mental Health Services Administration (SAMHSA, n.d.-a) website provides an Evidence-Based Practices Resource Center, which includes a broad spectrum of prevention and treatment options for substance use across the lifespan as well as a comprehensive listing of organizational websites related to EBP for substance use prevention, intervention, and treatment. Additionally, SAMHSA produces several EBP publications, including the Treatment Improvement Protocol (TIP), the Technical

Assistance Protocol (TAP), and the Treatment Advisory series, among others. These evidence-based documents are developed with the consensus of large and diverse groups of experts in the field and are readily available for free download from the SAMHSA Store website.

Systematic reviews and meta-analyses of scientific studies are among the highest levels of evidence to support professional practice. Examples of these can be found and reviewed at Cochrane and the Campbell Collaboration websites. Together with the Pan American Health Organization (PAHO) and World Health Organization (WHO), the Campbell Collaboration uses research data to inform decision-making related to substance use treatment and social determinants of health. Additionally, the Joanna Briggs Institute (2018), an international, not-for-profit research and development center, offers a wide range of research and education services regarding EBP for nursing, medicine, allied health, and information and health sciences.

Substance Use Across the Lifespan

Substance use negatively impacts all populations across the lifespan. Nurses provide direct care to individuals affected by substance use, including newborns, children, adolescents, adults, and older adult populations. The deleterious consequences of substance use, especially in light of the current opioid crisis, create an urgency for nurses in all generalist and specialty settings to take action.

MATERNAL AND CHILD HEALTH

Among women who use drugs, a majority of pregnancies are unintended. Once women are aware of the pregnancy, some, but not all, decrease or eliminate substance use.

In the United States, about one third of mothers who had live births reported mistimed or unwanted pregnancies, thus increasing the likelihood that substance use may be continued before pregnancy is detected (MacAfee et al., 2019).

Maternal cigarette smoking has been associated with preterm delivery, lower birth weights, and increased risk of sudden infant death syndrome (Centers for Disease Control and Prevention [CDC], 2020e). Nearly 20% of women report cigarette smoking in the three months before pregnancy; more than half of those women smoke through the third trimester of pregnancy (CDC, 2020b).

Over half of women consume alcohol within three months prior to the pregnancy, but this decreases to 8% who have any alcohol during the last trimester (CDC, 2020b).

In utero exposure to alcohol, especially during the first trimester, can cause miscarriage, stillbirth, and fetal alcohol spectrum disorders

(FASDs). Children with FASDs may have intellectual disabilities, physical abnormalities, and behavioral disabilities (CDC, 2020f).

From 1999 to 2014, the rate of opioid use disorder among pregnant women quadrupled (Haight et al., 2018). Potential consequences of opioid use during pregnancy include preterm birth, low birthweight, and maternal mortality (CDC, 2018c). Additionally, infants exposed to opioids prenatally may exhibit signs of neonatal abstinence syndrome (NAS). This syndrome is characterized by a range of withdrawal symptoms, including hyperactive reflexes, seizures, fever, dehydration, diarrhea, irritability, excessive crying, and difficulty being consoled. These symptoms may lead to poor feeding, failure to gain weight, and poor maternal–infant bonding (Wood et al., 2019).

YOUNG CHILDREN

Although substance use is possible among young children, older children are at a higher risk of developing substance use. Children are negatively impacted by family substance use. Those whose parents have a substance use disorder (SUD) are more likely to have lower socioeconomic status and have increased difficulty in academic, social, and family functioning. Children of parents with active substance use are at higher risk for experiencing abuse or neglect and of using substances themselves (Biederman et al., 2000; Lipari & Van Horn, 2017; Peleg-Oren & Teichman, 2006; Smit et al., 2020). Parental substance use is the second most common reason for removal from the home by protective services (Lipari & Van Horn, 2017).

ADOLESCENTS

Experimentation with substances, as well as onset of problematic use, may occur during adolescence, with tobacco, alcohol, and cannabis (marijuana) typically ranking high among substances used. According to results indicating current use of substances in the *2017 Youth Risk Behavior Surveillance* survey, nearly one third of high school students (29.8%) reported alcohol use; nearly 20% reported use of cannabis or some type of tobacco—cigarettes, cigars, or smokeless tobacco or electronic vapor product use (Kann et al., 2018).

Tobacco use typically starts and is established prior to age 18 (CDC, 2019b). According to the 2018 *Monitoring the Future* (MTF) survey, the rate of lifetime cigarette smoking prevalence was 23.8% by the 12th grade, and 30% reported vaping nicotine in the past year (Johnston et al., 2019). The risks related to smoking (e.g., cancer, cardiac disease, respiratory disease) have been well known for decades. The use of e-cigarettes and vaping has evolved more recently, particularly among adolescents, and its risks are beginning to emerge. In early 2020, the CDC, the U.S. Food and Drug Administration (FDA), state and local health departments, and other clinical and public health partners began investigating a national outbreak of e-cigarette, or vaping product, use-associated lung injury (EVALI; CDC, 2020c). These types of lung injuries commonly present as pneumonia, damage to alveoli, or an inflammatory reaction called fibrinous pneumonitis (Wolf & Rock, 2020). National and state data from patient reports and product sample testing showed that tetrahydrocannabinol (THC)-containing e-cigarette or vaping products, particularly from informal sources like friends, family, or in-person or online dealers, were linked to most EVALI cases and played a major role in the outbreak (CDC, 2020c).

Underage use of alcohol persists despite the minimum legal drinking age of 21 years in the United States. The rate of current alcohol use among 12–20-year-olds has remained steady at approximately 20% over the past few years (CDC, 2020a). Consequences of underage alcohol use include social problems, school failure or underachievement, legal issues, violence, use of other drugs, changes in brain development, and unintentional injuries (CDC, 2020a). Early use of alcohol is associated with higher rates of the onset of alcohol use disorders (SAMSHA, 2018). It is notable that alcohol use contributes to other risky behaviors, such as riding in cars with people who are drinking, which increases the likelihood of unintentional injury and traffic fatalities. Alcohol use also increases the risk for engaging in unsafe sexual behaviors. Among sexually active students, 18.8% drank alcohol or used drugs before their last instance of sexual intercourse (Kann et al., 2018), which increased their risks for unplanned pregnancy and infectious diseases.

Although any underage alcohol use is illegal and problematic, many youth engage in "binge drinking," which is even more hazardous.

According to the Youth Risk Behavior Surveillance System (YRBSS), 13.5% of surveyed students binge drank (4+ drinks if female, 5+ drinks if male) on one occasion during the past 30 days, and some youth (4.4%) reported drinking 10 or more drinks on one occasion (Kann et al., 2018). Deaths related to excessive alcohol are estimated at 4,300 underaged youths per year in the United States (CDC, 2020a).

Cannabis is widely used among youth. Results from the 2018 MTF survey indicate that the annual prevalence of cannabis use ranged from 11% to 36% in Grades 8, 10, and 12 (Johnston et al., 2019). These results are confirmed by the YRBSS, which indicated that 35.6% of high school students had ever used cannabis, and 19.8% were current users (Kann et al., 2018).

Cannabis consumption can cause perceptual alterations, cognitive disturbances, slowed responses, altered thought processes, and memory problems (National Institute on Drug Abuse [NIDA], 2020a). Over the past several decades, there have been notable increases in the potency of cannabis; the average level of tetrahydrocannabinoid (THC) was 3.8% in the 1990s, 12.2% in 2014, and up to 16% in 2018 (NIDA, 2020a). There is a dose-response relationship between cannabis use and an increased risk of psychotic disorders, including schizophrenia; the greatest risk of later psychosis is from high-potency cannabis and synthetic cannabinoids (Malone et al., 2010). With the growing popularity of vaping devices, teens have also started vaping THC; nearly 4% of 12th graders say they vape THC daily (NIDA, 2019).

The use of "hard" drugs such as heroin and cocaine among teens and young adults is less prevalent than alcohol and cannabis, although they bear more serious consequences. The YRBSS found that 4.8% of students had ever used cocaine, 1.7% had ever used heroin, and 1.5% had ever injected any illegal drugs. Other illicit drugs include, but are not limited to, synthetic cannabinoids, methamphetamines, hallucinogens, ecstasy/MDMA, and inhalants. Prescription drugs can also be misused (used illicitly). This remains a significant problem, as about 14% of students have used prescription pain medicines without a doctor's order or differently than prescribed (Kann et al., 2018).

ADULTS

About 10% of all adults in the United States have an underlying substance use disorder. People aged 18–25 have the highest prevalence of substance use for all categories, with 56.3% having had any alcohol use, 24.2% of people aged 18–25 having used any illicit drugs, and 22.1% having used cannabis. Among those aged 26 years and older, 55.8% had any alcohol use, 9.5% had used an illicit drug, and 7.9% had used cannabis (SAMHSA, 2018).

"Binge drinking" is defined by the National Institute on Alcohol Abuse and Alcoholism (NIAAA, n.d.) as a pattern of drinking that brings blood alcohol concentration (BAC) levels to 0.08 g/dL in about 2 hours, and by SAMHSA as 5 or more drinks for men or 4 or more drinks for women on the same occasion (i.e., at the same time or within a couple of hours of each other) on at least 1 day in the past month. "Heavy alcohol use" is defined by SAMHSA as binge drinking on 5 or more days in the past month. Among those Americans aged 18–25 who used alcohol, 36.9% reported binge drinking, and 9.6% reported heavy alcohol use. Among Americans aged 26 years and older, 24.7% reported binge drinking, and 6.2% had heavy alcohol use (SAMHSA, 2018). Alcohol use contributes to a broad range of serious health threats. The World Health Organization (WHO) estimates that in 2016, 3 million deaths globally were attributable to heavy alcohol use, largely due to digestive diseases, unintentional injuries, cardiovascular diseases, and diabetes (WHO, 2018).

Among adults, tobacco use has generally been declining over the past 5 decades, but it continues to be the leading cause of preventable death (CDC, 2020c). Health risks from tobacco use have long been known (e.g., it causes most cases of lung cancer). Smoking is connected with cancers throughout the body systems, COPD, emphysema, chronic bronchitis, and cardiovascular disease. It is a cause of stroke and coronary heart disease, among the leading causes of death in the United States (National Center for Chronic Disease Prevention and Health Promotion Office on Smoking and Health, 2014).

Cigarette smoking often accompanies illicit drug use, perhaps serving as a drug cue and relapse trigger. Many people who use tobacco also meet the criteria for an alcohol or drug use disorder or mental illness. Smoking may account for up to two thirds of the difference in life expectancy for those with serious behavioral health disorders (NIAAA, 2008; NIDA, 2018b; Tam et al., 2016).

Health implications associated with substance use, particularly as they relate to risks for transmission of infectious diseases and overdoses, largely depend on the specific type, quantity, and purity of the substance and the route of its administration. Drug overdose deaths affect all adult age groups. In 2017, drug overdoses were responsible for 70,237 deaths; 67.8% involved opioids (Scholl et al., 2019). Intravenous drug use is a leading cause of infectious diseases, including HIV/AIDS and hepatitis. While the incidence of HIV/AIDS was thought to be stabilizing for several years, in 2017, there was a spike in the number of people newly diagnosed with HIV, the majority of whom were under age 35 (CDC, 2020g). Other infectious diseases such as hepatitis C also increased, with acute cases in 20–29-year-olds, at a rate three times higher than the general population. The marked increase in infectious diseases was directly related to IV drug use and shared needles (Schillie et al., 2020).

ADULTS 65 AND OLDER

Substance use among older adults is a growing public health problem, especially as the baby boomer generation ages. Older adults are more likely than those in other age groups to have chronic health conditions and to take prescription medications. They are often prescribed medications for physical and psychological disorders or chronic pain that may interact with alcohol or other substances. Thus, substance use can cause more adverse effects and lead to more severe outcomes for older adults, largely due to comorbid conditions and age-related changes in metabolism.

Common causes of chronic pain among older adults include osteoarthritis, neuralgias, cancer, fibromyalgia, post-stroke pain, diabetic peripheral neuropathy and other chronic conditions (International Association for the Study of Pain, n.d.; Patel et al., 2014). Misuse of opioid pain medication is uncommon among older adults (Blazer & Wu, 2009), but opioid-related hospital admissions and emergency department visits are greatly increasing due to opioid overuse, dependence, poisoning, and adverse effects (Owens et al., 2014; Weiss et al., 2018). Like all other age groups, older adults have seen a sharp climb in overdose deaths over the past 2 decades. Among people aged 65 and older, the number of overdose deaths increased nearly four-fold from 1999 to 2017, suggesting an age-related vulnerability to opioids contributing to morbidity and mortality (CDC, 2018a).

Among other substances prevalent in this age group, alcohol is one of the most problematic. On any given day, 6 million adults aged 65 or older use alcohol, and about 978,000 have an alcohol use disorder. Adults 65 and older account for over 80% of deaths from falls related to alcohol use (CDC, n.d.). About 161,000 older adults have illicit substance use disorders (Mattson et al., 2017). Cannabis use has increased in this population, likely related to the aging baby boomer generation's prior experiences with cannabis and changes in societal views about and the legalization of recreational and medical cannabis use (Briscoe & Casarett, 2018; Kerr et al., 2017).

A comprehensive approach to patient safety for older adults aged 65 and over includes improved medication selection to reduce the risk of adverse drug events related to opioids, benzodiazepines, sleeping medications, and other medications with an unfavorable balance of benefits and harms. Normative age-related changes in metabolism, in conjunction with substance use or inappropriate use of prescribed medications can lead to neurotoxicity and other cognitive changes. The sedative effects of certain medications can contribute to drug-drug interactions, alcohol-drug interactions, an increased potential for falls and other accidents, and exacerbation of existing medical problems. Teaching older adults about these types of problems in a nonjudgmental manner using motivational communication techniques can be helpful for risk reduction and treatment access if indicated (Blow et al., 2020). Another important component of this safety strategy for clinicians involves use of the American Geriatrics Society (AGS) Beers Criteria® for potentially inappropriate medication (PIM) use in older adults (American Geriatrics Society Beers Criteria® Update Expert Panel, 2019).

Services in the Continuum of Care

There are four major service categories in a substance use disorder (SUD) services continuum of care, which refers to a comprehensive array of health services spanning all levels and intensity of care, delivered over a period of time. At one end of the continuum is prevention services, which are provided for individuals and populations who have not yet experienced the onset of disease (Center for Substance Abuse Prevention [CSAP], 2009, 2019). The next level in the care continuum is early intervention, which refers to detection (screening) and early provision of interventions to address identified problems, consistent with the Screening, Brief Intervention, and Referral to Treatment (SBIRT) model. The third category in the comprehensive continuum of care is specialty addictions treatment, which refers to a menu of treatment resources, which will be discussed later. The fourth category is ongoing continuing care and recovery support, including post-treatment monitoring and supportive services for all clients, not only those discharged successfully from treatment (Fornili, 2016a, 2016b).

PREVENTION

Substance use prevention activities are designed to educate and support individuals and communities to prevent the use and misuse of drugs and the development of SUDs (Substance Abuse and Mental Health Services Administration [SAMHSA], 2020c). Caplan, one of the first scholars in prevention psychiatry, provided conceptual definitions for primary, secondary, and tertiary prevention within a population-based public health context. He described primary prevention as activities to promote health before the onset of a disorder, secondary prevention as early diagnosis and treatment of existing cases, and tertiary prevention as the rehabilitation of individuals who are already suffering from a problem or disorder

(Caplan, 1964; Center for the Application of Prevention Technologies, n.d.; O'Connell et al., 2009). In 1983, Gordon proposed an alternative classification of prevention services focused on population health (universal, selective, and indicated prevention services).

According to Gordon's model, *universal* prevention strategies reduce the probability of a disorder among an entire population, *selective* prevention strategies are targeted to subpopulations at elevated risks for a disorder and *indicated* prevention strategies are for individuals who have been screened or identified as having increased vulnerability, asymptomatic illness, or both (Gordon, 1983; O'Connell et al., 2009). From a substance-related perspective, *universal* prevention services are delivered to entire populations (e.g., all school-aged children) to prevent initiation of substance use. *Selective* phase strategies are geared to subpopulations at known risk for substance use (such as children with family histories of substance use and/or child abuse), who have not yet initiated substance use but are at higher risk than the general population. *Indicated* strategies are more specifically aimed at members exhibiting risk that is linked to substance misuse. Members of this group are not formally diagnosed as having a SUD but are exhibiting risk factors that enhance their chance of developing substance use problems. They may, for example, have failing grades, exhibit estrangement from peers and parents, or be involved with the criminal justice system.

Inconsistent success in the prevention of substance misuse has necessitated a significant shift in how prevention services are delivered and how their outcomes are evaluated. The emphasis is now on surveillance of population-level data regarding substance use and consequences, and on the identification of risk and protective factors. This public health approach aims to target evidence-based, culturally relevant prevention services to individuals and groups within specific communities and subpopulation groups. It is assumed that reduction or elimination of risk factors and enhancement of protective factors contribute to long-term changes in thinking, feelings, and behaviors of individuals and communities (SAMHSA, 2019a). Renstrom et al. (2017) summarized information about shared risk and protective factors from the United Nations Office on Drugs and Crime (UNODC, 2013) and the European Monitoring

Centre for Drugs and Drug Addiction Best Practices Portal (EMCDDA, 2016). According to Renstrom et al. (p. 200), risk factors for substance use include the following:

- High availability
- Substance use/dependence among parents
- Substance use by older siblings
- Lack of parental supervision
- Low quality of family relations
- Family disruption and problematic economic conditions
- Low perception of harm in society, especially among young people
- Individual risk factors: mental disorder, conduct disorder, aggressive behavior, and academic failure

Protective factors to reduce or prevent substance use include the following:

- Reduced availability and high prices
- Parental monitoring
- Academic competence
- Effective policies
- Strong neighborhood attachment
- Strong positive attachment or bond between children and parents
- Positive external support system
- Individual attributes such as temperament and disposition, self-control (Renstrom et al., 2017, p. 200)

Within the U.S. Department of Health and Human Services, SAMHSA has identified prevention strategies with a track record of demonstrated success and categorized risk and protective factors according to three areas of influence:

- *Individual factors*, which include behavior and personality as well as genetic and physical make up;

- *Family factors*, which include the way that parents and children behave and relate to each other; and
- *Environmental factors*, which include circumstances outside of the family such as school experiences, peer influences, and community conditions (SAMHSA, 2019a).

Most strategies to address these factors are related to youth, although many are applicable to families across the lifespan. To maximize success and have the greatest impact, SAMHSA recognizes that prevention programs should reduce exposure to risks while enhancing protective factors, and build on strengths in the individual, family, and environment. It may be important to combine activities to address more than one risk factor at a time. Further, SAMHSA recommends focusing prevention efforts on young, school-aged children and their families before negative behaviors and family problems become deep-rooted. They also recommend choosing strategies that fit children's gender and level of development and developing prevention activities in more than one context, such as schools, cultural settings, faith-based groups, and neighborhoods (SAMHSA, 2019a).

Strategic Prevention Framework

The SAMHSA CSAP Strategic Prevention Framework (SPF) is a flexible, evidence-driven, comprehensive, community-based guide for planning strategies to address risk and protective factors (CSAP, 2009). It offers a structure for planning and designing programs to prevent and continually monitor substance misuse at the population and subpopulation levels (Figure 1). Community members participate at each of the five steps (assessment, capacity, planning, implementation, and evaluation) to ensure buy-in and an approach that maintains relevancy to the needs of the targeted population (SAMHSA, 2019a). Sustainability and cultural competence are key "cross-cutting" principles in the SPF framework.

The SPF is a planning model in which nurses and community stakeholders identify culturally appropriate, evidence-based prevention services to address specific needs in their communities. Part of the assessment phase entails ascertaining service and resource gaps, recognizing

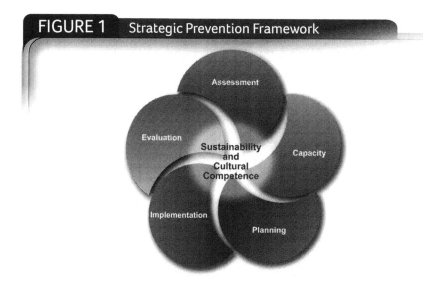

FIGURE 1 Strategic Prevention Framework

From *A Guide to SAMHSA's Strategic Prevention Framework* by Substance Abuse and Mental Health Services Administration, 2019a, June. Copyright 2019 by SAMHSA. Reprinted with permission.

community assets, and identifying risk factors germane to specific sub-populations. The next phase is program planning, wherein community members are involved in the selection of evidenced-based prevention and intervention strategies. Evaluation involves ongoing surveillance of process and outcome measures so that ineffective strategies can be replaced with more successful prevention services.

The SPF model is similar to the nursing process for population health, in that it involves assessment, planning, implementation, and evaluation. However, SPF adds a fifth step, capacity, which refers to building the availability and accessibility of resources and the readiness of communities to address prevention needs (SAMHSA, 2019a). The SPF model provides addictions nurses and other prevention services specialists a guide for working with a variety of community-based organizations, such as organized youth groups, faith-based groups, community service organizations (such as Lions, Rotary, and Kiwanis clubs), prison populations, and family groups. Sustainability and cultural competence are important concepts at the center of the SPF schematic. Sustainability refers to a process of securing steady funding streams and maintaining and evaluating a flexible, coordinated, effective, and enduring prevention services system. Cultural competence refers to the ability to be sensitive and communicate with diverse groups, which is essential to the success of community-based prevention programs. Prevention is embedded in contemporary nursing practice. Addictions nurses utilize evidence-based life span approaches for substance use prevention among diverse populations (CSAP, 2009; Bennett et al., 1983). Nurses in all settings (individual, group, family, and/or community) have abundant opportunities to assume essential roles in substance use prevention (Vourakis & Bennett, 1979).

EARLY INTERVENTION

Early intervention for substance-related problems in primary care and other healthcare settings rely most heavily on principles of early recognition (detection) and minimization of harm (Babor et al., 1986), especially among individuals who had not yet developed the need for extensive, specialized treatment (SAMHSA, 2013). Undetected or untreated SUDs are associated with other, often life-threatening, physical, mental health, and social conditions.

Screening, Brief Intervention, and Referral to Treatment

In 1990, the Institute of Medicine called for improved screening and detection of alcohol problems among non-treatment-seeking individuals receiving services within community-based agencies, including primary care provider offices. Subsequently, the WHO endorsed, supported, and replicated the development of initiatives for SUD early intervention (Babor & Higgins-Biddle, 2001; Babor et al., 2001; Saunders et al., 1993). These interventions have become known as SBIRT—the Screening, Brief Intervention, and Referral to Treatment model (SAMHSA, 2013).

Traditionally, treatment for alcohol problems has been delivered primarily in specialized institutions focused on individuals with more advanced disorders but not on individuals with harmful/hazardous use (Babor et al., 1986). SBIRT has become recognized for its suitability in any healthcare setting, especially for the identification of SUD at early stages of disease (SAMHSA, 2013). It includes screening with standardized, validated instruments, engaging lower risk patients in short conversations about their substance use behaviors, and referring patients with higher risks for comprehensive assessments and SUD treatment if indicated (SAMHSA, 2013).

Millions of Americans need but do not receive treatment (Park-Lee et al., 2017). Early identification through screening and brief intervention, coupled with facilitated referrals to treatment can reduce the "treatment gap" and improve the health of individuals, families, and communities. Despite more than 5 decades of evidence in support of this practice, SBIRT remains underimplemented in many settings (Saitz, 2007). There is strong evidence in the literature that screening and brief counseling interventions are effective in detecting alcohol problems and decreasing alcohol consumption among adult patients in primary care settings (Moyer & U.S. Preventive Services Task Force, 2013), although evidence is somewhat weaker regarding screening for drug problems among primary care patients (Polen et al., 2008). Many people who consume unhealthy amounts of alcohol are more likely to use illicit drugs (Kurti et al., 2016), and should also be asked about their drug use (Smith et al., 2014). An unstructured approach in which clinicians ask questions about substance use whenever they deem it relevant may detect more patients with higher problem severity; however, systematic (universal) screening with standardized instruments may detect more patients overall and more patients at lower levels of risk. These findings suggest that universal screening may be more effective in detecting substance problems at earlier stages of disease (Reinholdz et al., 2013).

Utilization of SBIRT for the early detection of alcohol, tobacco, and other drug use has been endorsed by numerous governmental organizations, including the Joint Commission (2014), the National Quality Forum (2014), the National Institute on Alcohol Abuse and Alcoholism (NIAAA, 2007), and the National Institute on Drug Abuse (NIDA).

Many professional organizations have also endorsed SBIRT, including the International Nurses Society on Addictions (IntNSA), and the Emergency Nurses Association (ENA) recently updated a joint position paper calling for nurses in all specialties and practice settings to deliver SBIRT (Schieferle et al., 2020).

Numerous substance screening tools exist, but the Alcohol Use Disorder Identification Test (AUDIT) has high degrees of sensitivity (99%) and good specificity (74%), making it effective in differentiating those with and without an alcohol use disorder (AUD; Babor et al., 2001; Rubinsky et al., 2010). It is useful for early intervention because it can detect heavy drinking as well as serious AUD (Bush et al., 1998). The Readiness Ruler can be utilized to determine the individual's level of readiness and intention to change their substance use behaviors. Some Readiness Rulers can also be used to inquire about use of multiple substances in addition to alcohol (Heather et al., 2008). It is also helpful to incorporate screening for underlying psychiatric conditions, which may increase problem severity and the complexity of treatment required.

Brief interventions are effective, and encouraged, for individuals who have harmful or hazardous alcohol use (e.g., those that exceed NIAAA recommendations for frequency and quantity of alcohol consumption) but who have not yet developed severe alcohol disorders (NIAAA, 2007). However, brief interventions may be insufficient for people who use or misuse drugs, or who have more complex and severe alcohol or drug disorders as well as those with co-occurring psychiatric disorders (Roy-Byrne et al., 2014; Saitz et al., 2014; SAMHSA, 2013). For these individuals, *specialty treatment* is indicated.

Facilitated referrals to treatment are a distinguishing feature of a comprehensive, integrated SBIRT model. SBIRT providers in generalist settings (e.g., primary care, emergency services) are encouraged to have prearranged relationships with specialty treatment providers in order to initiate and facilitate referrals (SAMHSA, 2013). Specialty SUD treatment is effective, especially when patients are satisfied that their care is of sufficient quantity, quality, and service intensity (Hser et al., 2014).

The Recovery Management (RM) model, situated within a larger Recovery-Oriented Systems of Care model (White, 2008), can help to conceptually explain relationships between a recovery-oriented care continuum and components of SBIRT (Fornili, 2016a, 2016b). A recovery-oriented SUD care continuum includes prevention, early intervention, specialty treatment, and continuing care services. Key RM model concepts include prerecovery identification and engagement, recovery initiation and stabilization, sustained recovery support, and long-term recovery maintenance (White, 2008). Within a recovery-oriented care continuum (Figure 2), *prerecovery identification* corresponds to the screening and brief intervention (SBI) components of SBIRT, and *recovery initiation and stabilization* corresponds to the referral to treatment (RT) component of SBIRT.

Two remaining RM concepts in the SBIRT Plus RM model are absent from traditional SBIRT models. These are *sustained recovery support* and *long-term recovery maintenance*. The SBIRT Plus RM model highlights additional roles and responsibilities for generalist care providers beyond the referral component of SBIRT. A recovery-oriented SBIRT model

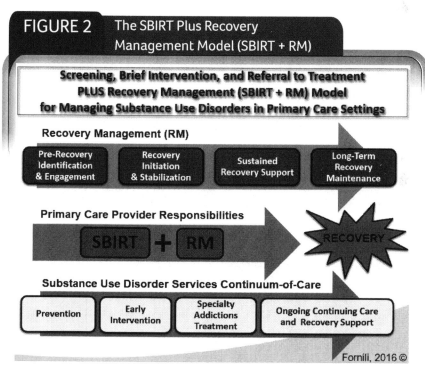

From "Part 2: Screening, Brief Intervention, and Referral to Treatment Plus Recovery Management," by K. Fornili, 2016b, *Journal of Addictions Nursing*, 27(2), p. 87. Copyright 2016 by Fornili. Reprinted with permission.

should include ongoing monitoring, encouragement, and support; care coordination; medication management; post-treatment "recovery check-ups"; and facilitated reentry to specialty treatment if indicated (Fornili, 2016b; White, 2008).

MULTIDIMENSIONAL ASSESSMENT AND TREATMENT PLANNING

A comprehensive, multidimensional, biopsychosocial assessment is performed in order to identify the individual's risks, needs, strengths, skills, and resources. An individualized treatment plan is developed to address all aspects of a person's life (ASAM, 2015). Resulting services may encompass pretreatment, treatment, continuing care, and support throughout recovery. Medical, mental health, and other follow-up services (e.g., community- or family-based recovery support systems) are also crucial to a person's success in achieving and maintaining recovery. Behavioral therapies are necessary to help patients modify their attitudes and beliefs about their disorders and support appropriate behavioral change. Medications may augment treatment adherence by reducing cravings and stabilizing mood (NIDA, 2019). Goals are to sustain involvement in treatment and help the patient to develop healthy life skills.

American Society of Addiction Medicine Treatment Criteria for Addictive, Substance-Related, and Co-occurring Conditions

Comprehensive, multidimensional assessment and standardized placement criteria help to match an individual's specific treatment needs and problem severity to an appropriate level of care that best ensures their safety and promotes recovery in all life domains.

The American Society of Addiction Medicine's *ASAM Criteria* is a widely used and comprehensive set of guidelines for placement, continued stay, and transfer and discharge of patients with addiction and co-occurring conditions (Mee-Lee et al., 2013). *ASAM Criteria* defines treatment as a continuum of care marked by four broad levels of service and an early intervention level. Within these five levels, decimal numbers are used to further express gradations of intensity of services. These levels of care provide a standard nomenclature for describing the continuum of recovery-oriented addiction services and provide clinicians with a recommended level of care that matches the intensity of treatment services to identified patient needs.

ASAM Levels of Care

See the brief descriptions for each ASAM level of care. More detailed descriptions of these services, based on an ASAM multidimensional needs assessment, can be found in *The ASAM Criteria: Treatment Criteria for Addictive, Substance-Related, and Co-occurring Conditions* (Mee-Lee et al., 2013) and *The ASAM Essentials of Addiction Medicine*, 3rd Edition (Mee-Lee & Shulman, 2020):

- *ASAM Level 0.5*—Early Intervention for Adults and Adolescents: This service is for individuals who are at risk of developing substance-related problems or for whom there is insufficient information to document a diagnosable SUD. The SBIRT model falls under this level of care.
- *ASAM Level 1*—Outpatient Services for Adults and Adolescents: This level of care typically consists of less than 9 hours of service per week for adults, or less than 6 hours per week for adolescents. It consists of recovery or motivational enhancement therapies and strategies and encompasses organized services that may be delivered in a wide variety of settings.
- *ASAM Level 2.1*—Intensive Outpatient (IOP) Services for Adults and Adolescents: This level of care typically is used to treat multidimensional instability and consists of 9 or more hours of service per week for adults, or 6 or more hours per week for adolescents. To accommodate the patient's need to work or attend school, it can be delivered during the day, before or after work or school, in the evening, and/or on weekends.
- *ASAM Level 2.5*—Partial Hospitalization Services for Adults and Adolescents: This level of care typically provides 20 or more hours of service per week for multidimensional instability that

does not require 24-hour care. These services are capable of meeting the complex needs of people with addiction and co-occurring conditions.

- *ASAM Level 3.1*—Clinically Managed Low-Intensity Residential Services for Adults and Adolescents: Level 3 "clinically managed" care places emphasis on the therapeutic milieu for individuals with minimal problems with intoxication and withdrawal or medical complications. Levels 3.1–3.5 encompass co-occurring capable, co-occurring enhanced, and complexity capable residential services, staffed by addictions, mental health, and general medical personnel. Level 3.1 typically provides living support and structure 24-hours per day and at least 5 hours of low-intensity treatment for SUD per week.
- *ASAM Level 3.3*—Clinically Managed Population-Specific High-Intensity Residential Services (Adults only): This level of care typically offers 24-hour care with trained counselors to stabilize multidimensional imminent danger. This level provides a less intense milieu and group treatment for patients with cognitive or other impairments who are unable to use a full active milieu or therapeutic community.
- *ASAM Level 3.5*—Clinically Managed Medium-Intensity Residential Services for Adolescents and Clinically Managed High-Intensity Residential Services for Adults: This level of care offers 24-hour care with trained counselors to stabilize multidimensional imminent danger and prepare patients for outpatient treatment. Patients in this level are able to use a full active milieu or therapeutic community.
- *ASAM Level 3.7*—Medically Monitored High-Intensity Inpatient Services for Adolescents and Medically Monitored High-Intensity Inpatient Services for Adults: This level of care provides 24-hour nursing care with physician availability for significant problems in acute intoxication and/or withdrawal potential; biomedical conditions and complications; and emotional, behavioral, or cognitive conditions and complications. Patients in this level of care require medication and have a recent history of past and current inability to complete withdrawal management and enter

into continuing addiction treatment. This is the appropriate setting for patients with subacute biomedical and emotional, behavioral, or cognitive problems that are so severe that they require inpatient treatment.

- *ASAM Level 4.0*—Medically Managed Intensive Inpatient Services for Adolescents and Adults: This level of care provides 24-hour nursing care and daily physician care for severe, unstable problems in acute intoxication and/or withdrawal potential; biomedical conditions and complications; and emotional, behavioral, or cognitive conditions and complications.
- Opioid Treatment Program (OTP): In this level of care, opioid medication is provided daily or several times per week, and counseling is available to maintain multidimensional stability for those with opioid use disorder (OUD).

OTPs (formerly referred to as "methadone clinics") provide a range of services to reduce, eliminate, or prevent the use of illicit drugs, potential criminal activity, and/or the spread of infectious disease. Their focus is on helping the individual receiving medications for the treatment of OUDs achieve and sustain recovery and improve their quality of life. OTPs must be certified by SAMHSA and accredited by a SAMHSA-approved accrediting body. The Division of Pharmacologic Therapies (DPT), part of the SAMHSA Center for Substance Abuse Treatment (CSAT), oversees accreditation standards and certification processes for OTPs. Federal law requires patients who receive treatment in an OTP to receive medical, counseling, vocational, educational, and other assessment and treatment services, in addition to prescribed medication. As of 2020, OTPs are located in every U.S. state and territory except Wyoming and Guam (SAMHSA, 2020f).

MEDICATIONS FOR THE TREATMENT OF SUBSTANCE USE DISORDERS

The use of medications along with behavioral therapies provides a "whole-patient" approach that helps patients achieve and sustain recovery. Medications for the treatment of SUD can help normalize brain chemistry, block the euphoric effects of alcohol, tobacco, and opioids, relieve physiological cravings, and normalize body functions without the negative effects of the substance. Medications used for the treatment of SUD must be approved by the U.S. Food and Drug Administration (FDA) for this indication, and treatment programs that utilize these medications are clinically driven and tailored to meet each patient's needs (SAMHSA, 2020f). The ultimate goal for the use of these medications is full recovery, including the ability to live a self-directed life. This treatment approach has been shown to:

- Improve patient survival,
- Increase retention in treatment,
- Reduce the potential for relapse,
- Lower a person's risk of contracting infectious diseases like HIV or hepatitis,
- Decrease illicit opiate use and other criminal activity among people with SUD,
- Increase patients' ability to gain and maintain employment, and
- Improve birth outcomes among women who have SUD and are pregnant (SAMHSA, 2020f).

Unfortunately, medications for the treatment of SUD are greatly underused. The slow adoption of these evidence-based treatment options for alcohol and opioid dependence is partly due to misconceptions about substituting one drug for another. Discrimination against patients being treated with medications is also a factor, despite state and federal laws clearly prohibiting it. Other factors include lack of training for prescribers (physicians, advanced practice registered nurses, and physician assistants) and negative opinions toward medications for SUD. Addictions nurses responsible for assessing, monitoring, and evaluating the patient's responses to these medications can support the efforts of the individual to achieve long-lasting recovery.

Medications for Opioid Use Disorder and Opioid Overdose

Healthcare professionals should consider pharmacotherapy with all patients with OUD. There are three FDA-approved medications for the treatment of OUD, including the mu-opioid receptor full agonist methadone, the mu-opioid receptor partial agonist buprenorphine, and the mu-opioid receptor antagonists naltrexone and naloxone. Medications for OUD reduce illicit opioid use, retain people in treatment, and reduce the risk of overdose deaths better than treatment without medications. Stabilized patients that are taking medications for OUD are considered to be in recovery (SAMHSA, 2020e, 2020f):

- *Methadone* is the most studied medication for OUD. It has the oldest evidence base of all treatment approaches to OUD and has been in use for approximately 50 years. Methadone reduces opioid cravings and withdrawal and blunts or blocks the effects of illicit opioids. Numerous studies have shown that methadone treatment is associated with higher rates of treatment retention, and lower rates of illicit opioid use, mortality, criminal behavior, and HIV seroconversion. Administering and dispensing methadone for the treatment of OUD is limited to federally certified, accredited OTPs, formerly referred to as "methadone clinics" (SAMHSA, 2020e, 2020f).
- *Buprenorphine* (monotherapeutic agent) and *buprenorphine/ naloxone* (combination product), like methadone, have demonstrated efficacy compared to treatment without medications. However, unlike methadone, buprenorphine products can be prescribed in primary care or other office-based settings (as well as OTPs) by qualified practitioners with a waiver from SAMHSA's Center for Substance Abuse Treatment Division of Pharmacologic Therapies website (SAMHSA, 2022a).
- *Extended-release naltrexone* (XR-NTX) is FDA approved to prevent relapse in patients who have remained opioid abstinent for sufficient time. Pharmacotherapy for OUD should be accompanied by individually tailored medical management and psychosocial and recovery support services as needed and wanted by patients to support their recovery (SAMHSA, 2020e, 2020f).
- *Naloxone* is a lifesaving medication used for reversal of respiratory depression caused by heroin, morphine, or other opioid overdoses. In many states, naloxone is available without

prescription in local pharmacies as a nasal or an injectable medication. It is recommended that everyone who uses opioids, as well as a family member or friend, should have naloxone on hand to deal with emergencies such as depressed respiration, excessive sleepiness, and unresponsiveness. Individuals whose opioid overdoses are reversed in community settings with naloxone should be taken to an emergency department right away, due to naloxone's short half-life, the widespread use of long-acting opioids, and a high potential for return to an overdose state.

Medications for Alcohol Use Disorder

Currently, there are three FDA-approved medications for the treatment of alcohol use disorder (AUD). Disulfiram (Antabuse) works by increasing the concentration of acetaldehyde, a toxic byproduct that occurs when alcohol is metabolized. Because it causes a negative ("aversive") reaction when an individual uses small amounts of alcohol, the anticipation of unpleasant symptoms (nausea and flushing of the skin), can help some individuals avoid returning to alcohol use. Naltrexone (oral medication Revia® and injectable medication Vivitrol®) blocks opioid receptors, decreases pleasant sensations associated with drinking, and can reduce alcohol craving. Acamprosate (Campral®) is thought to ease negative effects of alcohol cessation by dampening glutamate activity and reducing hyperexcitability of the brain (NIAAA, 2019; SAMHSA, 2020f). Other medications that have shown promise in reducing alcohol consumption are not yet approved by the FDA.

Medications for Tobacco Use Disorder

There are two different types of medication for the treatment of nicotine dependence. The most widely known is nicotine replacement therapy (NRT), in which small, controlled amounts of nicotine are delivered in various forms (patches, gums, sprays) to satisfy cravings for nicotine without exposure to the dangerous chemicals found in cigarettes. The individual can then taper down the amount of nicotine they consume over time. Multiple over-the-counter NRT preparations are available for purchase in stores and pharmacies; some may be covered by health insurance or government programs at low to no cost. Non-nicotine prescription medications include varenicline (Chantix), which blocks nicotinic receptors, and bupropion (Zyban), which seems to inhibit the reuptake of norepinephrine and dopamine while acting to a lesser degree on nicotinic receptors. Zyban has been approved for smoking cessation, whereas the Wellbutrin formulation of bupropion is used for the management of depression. Medications for nicotine dependence help with nicotine withdrawal and cravings, but for maximum benefit, they should be combined with behavioral counseling, assistance in developing a quit plan, and for some people, peer support or professional coaching, which can be accessed through telephone smoking cessation quitlines.

DRUG TESTING IN CLINICAL PRACTICE

Drug testing is a therapeutic tool in evidence-based SUD treatment, as it assists providers to comprehensively assess patients' denial, motivation, adherence, drug use behaviors, and recovery outcomes. Clinical drug testing improves the objectivity of patient self-reports regarding use of specific controlled substances. It can also be helpful in assessing the chemical composition of illicit or nonprescribed substance(s) patients may have used and the timeframe in which they were ingested. Testing is not intended to be punitive; it may be helpful in deterring unauthorized use of substances and promoting adherence with prescribed treatment medications (e.g., methadone, buprenorphine). Drug testing results that contradict the patient's self-reported drug use are most appropriately addressed within the context of therapeutic discussions that promote motivation and reinforce abstinence (ASAM, 2017).

It is important to note that a positive drug screen (one that indicates the presence of a substance) provides insufficient information for diagnosing a SUD. Clinical drug screening should only be used in combination with other information. This includes information gleaned from nonjudgmental, nonconfrontational conversations with patients, physical and psychiatric examinations, medication reconciliations, and reports from prescription drug monitoring program (PDMP) databases (Reisfield et al., 2020). Addictions nurses should be aware of the advantages and disadvantages of each specific test, including its sensitivity and specificity (propensity for false negatives or false positives), the temporal component (e.g., the window of time for each substance included in the assay), cutoff values, and the potential for adulteration and contamination (ASAM, 2017).

As patient advocates, nurses need to have a clear understanding of the ultimate purpose for drug testing. Patients being monitored because of safety-sensitive occupations (e.g., nurses, commercial drivers, airplane pilots) or who are involved in the criminal justice system may be obligated to provide specimens for mandatory testing purposes. Monitoring and alternative programs may mandate that nurses and other healthcare providers with SUDs complete random drug testing as a monitoring requirement or for resumption of professional licenses. As an objective tool, drug testing can provide documentation for employers or regulators who require adherence to a treatment contract and abstinence from drug use.

RECOVERY SUPPORT AND CONTINUING CARE

A massive systems transformation has been underway for many years at the national, state, and local levels. The Recovery-Oriented Systems of Care (ROSC) model represents a broad conceptual shift in the addictions field, from a traditional focus on acute pathology and intervention to a focus on long-term personal and family recovery (White, 2008). Dennis et al. (2005) recognized that recovery is a journey, not an event, and that it takes about 5 years before recovery can be regarded as self-sustaining (Cano et al., 2017; Dennis et al., 2005). Recovery from alcohol and drug addiction, as endorsed by the U.S. Department of Health and Human Services SAMHSA, with the consensus of expert leaders and individuals in recovery, is defined as "a process of change through which people improve their health and wellness, live self-directed lives, and strive to reach their full potential" (SAMHSA, 2020d, para. 1).

Recovery is a journey that involves the growth of "recovery capital." Recovery capital refers to "the sum of resources that an individual can draw on to support their recovery pathway," (Cano et al., 2017, p. 11) including *personal capital* (i.e., self-esteem, resilience), *social capital* (i.e., networks and supports), and *community capital* (i.e., local housing, training, and employment resources). Strength-based treatment and support services that focus on the growth of recovery capital can maximize treatment outcomes (Cano et al., 2017).

SUDs have traditionally been treated like acute care illnesses. However, like hypertension, diabetes, and asthma, SUDs are chronic illnesses that require lifelong continuing care (McLellan et al., 2000). Treatment for all chronic medical conditions depends heavily on adherence to the treatment regimen. Adherence and relapse rates are similar across these chronic illnesses, including SUDs. Adherence and resulting outcomes are poorest among patients with inadequate social support, significant psychiatric comorbidity, and low socioeconomic status (McLellan et al., 2000). In a recovery-oriented system of care, health insurers and treatment providers deliver the same level of coverage and services for people with SUDs that they do for those receiving medical and surgical care. Outcomes and quality of life improve for patients with SUDs when parity in coverage and services exists.

Recovery Management (RM) provides a philosophical framework for organizing addictions treatment services to provide a continuum of quality-of-life enhancements for individuals and families affected by severe SUDs and extends addictions treatment from an acute care model to one of sustained recovery management. Key recovery-focused concepts of the RM model include prerecovery identification and engagement, recovery initiation and stabilization, sustained recovery support, and long-term recovery maintenance (White, 2008):

- *PreRecovery Identification and Engagement*: This RM concept is consistent with the screening and early identification components of SBIRT in primary care settings before the development of serious disorders (see Figure 2 and the earlier section on SBIRT): "The gradual onset and prolonged course of most severe substance use disorders provide windows of opportunity for screening and early intervention" (White, 2008, p. 53).

Prerecovery identification and engagement typically occurs in nonspecialized (non-SUD) community-based service settings, particularly primary healthcare settings. Engagement, on the part of the provider, refers to forming a therapeutic alliance with the patient, as well as awareness that a window of opportunity to intervene has become available. Engagement, on the part of the client, refers to a perceived belief that the provider is helpful and supportive (Fornili, 2016b).

Goals for prerecovery identification and engagement are to (a) identify and assess the magnitude of an individual's risk for future development of a SUD, (b) help at-risk individuals prevent or delay the onset of SUDs, (c) encourage the development of problem-solving and self-management strategies at early stages of problem development, (d) provide professional support to facilitate the resolution of early-stage problems, and (e) refer and assertively link individuals with more advanced problems to further professional assessment and the potential provision of specialized treatment and recovery support services (White, 2008).

- *Recovery Initiation and Stabilization*: Identification and referral are important first steps, but they do not routinely lead patients to initiate treatment. It is important that healthcare providers also provide supportive services to ensure that individuals with SUDs overcome barriers to care and actually initiate treatment (Garnick et al., 2009). Treatment can play a critical role in recovery initiation, but factors outside the treatment experience (e.g., family, peer support) are also critical (White, 2008). Recovery initiation occurs when a brief intervention leads to decreased alcohol (or drug) consumption and related risks and consequences. Recovery is also initiated when an individual accomplishes the steps necessary to access treatment so that they can begin the process of recovery at a level of specialty treatment matched to their individualized treatment needs (Fornili, 2016b). Individuals who do not access or complete treatment are those who are in greatest need of such treatment (White, 2008). Promising practices in enhancing engagement, retention, and stabilization include motivational interviewing (MI), expanding client decision-making, increasing one's focus on the development of the therapeutic alliance, and monitoring patient engagement. According to William White (2008), the earlier the initiation of treatment, the greater the level of recovery capital available to aid the transition from recovery initiation to stable, long-term recovery.

- *Sustained Recovery Support*: The RM model calls for transforming the provider relationship from one in which the provider is "an expert," to one in which the provider and the patient form a therapeutic alliance for long-term recovery support (White, 2008). In sustained recovery support, the emphasis is on the word "sustained." Recovery support services (RSS) are nonclinical services offered before, during, or in lieu of treatment; they may be delivered by nurses and other professionals (like primary care providers) as well as family members and peers in recovery. They may occur in a variety of community, faith-based, treatment, or other settings and are best delivered over a sustained period. The RSS continuum includes childcare, transportation, housing, life skills training, employment readiness, legal consultation, wellness checks, and self-management support (White, 2008).

- *Long-Term Recovery Maintenance*: Traditionally, addiction treatment services have been institution based, with service providers typically having little or no contact with the natural environments of patients and their families. Long-term recovery maintenance involves shifting the focus from the clinical environment to the patient's natural environment (e.g., their homes, families, and communities; White, 2008). Patients and their families benefit from extended post-treatment monitoring and support, in which care is provided beyond the cycle of crisis intervention, symptom suppression, and hospitalization. In the RM model, sustained recovery enhancement includes providing patient education about recovery self-care, post-treatment recovery checkups, the use of community resources to support sustained recovery, and prompt reentry into treatment as needed (White, 2008).

MOTIVATIONAL INTERVIEWING

Motivation is key to substance use behavior change. Motivational interviewing (MI) is the most widely researched and disseminated counseling approach in SUD treatment. This technique is also often used as a therapeutic approach when implementing brief interventions for substance misuse in the SBIRT model. MI is a philosophical approach to working with patients as much as it is a therapeutic technique. Created by William Miller and Stephen Rollnick (1991), MI incorporates Rodgerian principles of positive regard for the individual in exploring and resolving ambivalence toward change.

Relationships, connections, partnerships, and engagement form the foundation of MI. Therapeutic alliances are developed during the engagement phase, which is a process wherein the clinician and the individual establish a mutually trusting and respectful helping relationship (Miller & Rollnick, 2013). Many people do not have a well-developed sense of self-efficacy and find it hard to believe that they can make or maintain behavior change. Improving self-efficacy (confidence in one's ability) may be one of the ways that MI promotes behavior change (Chariyeva et al., 2013). Improving self-efficacy elicits confidence, hope, and optimism that change is possible. Thus, MI is effective in producing positive outcomes of treatment, including higher rates of treatment completion, reductions in substance use following treatment, and a greater desire to stop the use of substances (SAMHSA, 2019b).

The spirit of MI (i.e., partnership, acceptance, compassion, and evocation) includes the core counseling skills required for enhancing an individual's motivation to change. These counseling skills are described in the acronym OARS—Open-ended questions, Affirmations, Reflective listening, and Summarization (SAMHSA, 2019b). Open-ended questions are key to the information-gathering process, set the tone for nonjudgmental exploration of the client's problems, and lead to collaborative problem-solving. Affirmations are statements of appreciation for the client, and their strengths, talents, and aspirations. Reflective listening promotes engagement, while poor listening skills make the client feel misunderstood, which leads to disengagement. Summaries are special applications of reflective listening intended to connect multiple ideas. These skills are used to elicit and reinforce change talk and help the individual more forward.

HARM REDUCTION SERVICES

Harm reduction is an important public health strategy for reducing morbidity and mortality among individuals who are continuing substance use and are not ready for or do not desire abstinence. The primary goal of harm reduction is to reduce the *effects* of problematic health behaviors without necessarily extinguishing the behaviors completely (Hawk et al., 2017). Harm reduction strategies are intended to prevent additional problems or deterioration among those who already have an active addictive problem, and therefore they can be classified as prevention interventions (DiClemente, 2006).

According to the transtheoretical model of change (DiClemente, 2006; Prochaska & DiClemente, 1982), individuals in the early stages of change may not yet be willing to quit their substance use. However, when exploring options to reduce the harm of substance use, an individual who is not ready for abstinence may be willing to alter *how* they use. Examples of harm reduction for alcohol use would include not driving while drinking, consuming water in between each alcoholic beverage, or setting goals for frequency and quantity limits. Harm reduction for intravenous drug use may include efforts to reduce the risk of overdose (only injecting drugs at a safe injection site or carrying naloxone) and to prevent the spread of HIV and hepatitis (using a needle exchange program). While engaging in efforts to reduce harm, individuals remain in contact with the health professionals who can engage them in treatment when they are ready.

Humanism is a fundamental harm reduction principle. Its emphasis is on valuing, caring for, respecting, and dignifying patients as individuals, with an acknowledgment that holding moral judgments against patients is counterproductive to positive health outcomes (Hawk et al., 2017). Incrementalism is another fundamental principle, in which any positive change is viewed as a step toward improved health. Practitioners who utilize harm reduction models are pragmatic, in that they continue to support the patient, with an understanding that abstinence may not be the patient's priority goal and that perfect health behaviors are rarely achieved.

Harm reduction models are based in individualism, in which each person has unique needs as well as strengths and may present along a spectrum of harms, needs, strengths, and receptivity. Harm reduction values autonomy, which is exemplified by an understanding that individuals ultimately make and are responsible for their own choices about their health risks and behaviors. The addictions nurse understands the role of a therapeutic, reciprocal alliance, and individualized patient-centered care. Thus, the nurse does not "fire" patients for not achieving abstinence or other health goals but rather helps patients to understand the impact of their choices (Hawk et al., 2017).

RELAPSE PREVENTION

Relapse is defined by ASAM as "a process in which an individual who has established abstinence or sobriety experiences recurrence of signs and symptoms of active addiction, often including resumption of the pathological pursuit of reward and/or relief through the use of substances and other behaviors" (Mee-Lee et al., 2013, p. 427). Exposure to rewarding substances and behaviors, environmental cues, or emotional stressors can trigger relapse (Mee-Lee et al., 2013). Developed as a behavioral maintenance program for the addictions treatment, relapse prevention (RP) is a cognitive-behavioral, self-management program that combines behavioral skill training, cognitive interventions, and lifestyle change procedures. It was designed to help individuals who are trying to maintain behavioral changes to anticipate and cope with the problem of relapse (Marlatt, 1985). RP can enhance recovery when included as a component of a multimodal treatment approach, especially in the context of continuing care (Douaihy et al., 2020). The main tenets of the RP model include *intrapersonal determinants* (self-efficacy, positive outcome expectancy, motivation for positive behavior change, effective coping strategies for dealing with high-risk situations, management of negative emotional states). Functional social support, especially support from people who do not use substances, is an *interpersonal determinant* that is predictive of long-term recovery. Effective RP strategies include helping people learn to identify early relapse warning signs and develop effective coping for use in high-risk situations. Other effective RP strategies include helping individuals identify and manage cravings and cues, challenge cognitive distortions, work toward a more balanced lifestyle, and adhere to behavior and medication treatment. These strategies can be incorporated into all modalities within the care continuum (Douaihy et al., 2020).

SELF-HELP AND MUTUAL SUPPORT

Addictions nurses recognize the benefits of mutual support groups and can convey the potential gains from participation to their patients, to nurses in other specialties, and to other healthcare team members. Mutual support groups, including twelve-step programs, represent a readily available resource for individuals with SUDs.

Mutual support groups are nonprofessional groups comprising members who share the same problem and voluntarily support one another in the recovery from that problem (Humphreys, 2004; CSAT, 2008).

Twelve-step groups such as Alcoholics Anonymous (aa.org) and Narcotics Anonymous (na.org) emphasize abstinence and have 12 core developmental steps to recovering from dependence (CSAT, 2008). Participants in twelve-step programs often maintain close supportive relationships with their sponsors, who are members in long-term recovery. Emphasis is on taking responsibility for one's own recovery, sharing personal narratives, helping others, recognizing and incorporating the existence of a "higher power" into one's daily life, and focusing on spiritual practices and beliefs. The spiritual component of twelve-step programs may help people attribute different meanings to stressful events or life experiences and mobilize additional motivation and behavioral coping skills. Twelve-step participation may predict improved substance use outcomes. These programs have demonstrated considerable effectiveness in helping people with SUD achieve and maintain abstinence and improve their overall psychosocial functioning and recovery (Donovan & Floyd, 2008; Kelly et al., 2011).

Although twelve-step fellowships are often perceived as *treatment*, they are more appropriately considered an *adjunct to treatment*. They do not provide many important components of effective, evidence-based care (NIDA, 2018a). Nurses should distinguish between professional treatment and self-help (American Academy of Addiction Psychiatry [AAAP], 2015). According to the AAAP, "treatment" involves a provider who takes professional responsibility for the individual's overall care. They provide a thorough evaluation, which includes diagnosing the severity of the disorder, assessing for co-occurring medical and psychiatric disorders as well as social problems, and developing an individualized treatment plan guided by professionally accepted practice guidelines (AAAP, 2015). A recovery-oriented treatment philosophy is critical for post-treatment recovery support and attainment of optimal outcomes. The designated provider is responsible for referring the individual for additional treatment or social services as needed; monitoring the individual's response to treatment over time; and continuing with therapeutic contact, whenever possible, until stable recovery has been attained (AAAP, 2015; White, 2008).

Language, Stigma, and Culturally Congruent Practice

COMMON GLOBAL LANGUAGE FOR ADDICTIONS AND ADDICTIONS NURSING

Attaining consensus on nomenclature, from nursing titles to diagnostic terminology used in day-to-day clinical practice, is essential for advancing the professional specialty within the United States and globally. Generally, it is believed that language used in describing problematic alcohol or substance use is a product of policy and attitudes toward the use of these substances. Despite calls for consensus on common terminology, variations based on geographical region or discipline remain (Kelly et al., 2016). It is essential to recognize how these variations may hinder understanding and why advocacy, policy, and collaborative efforts are needed for improved communication.

Perhaps the largest global challenge with the wide variety of terms relating to the core profession of addictions nursing is that nurses performing relatively similar clinical duties describe themselves differently. This may lead to a fragmented global professional identity and difficulties in advocating as a specialist group.

Some regions of the world use terms such as "substance abuse nurse" as opposed to "addictions nurse." Since "dependence" is closely aligned with the biochemical model of addiction, it is likely to be more accepted in medical settings, and some nurses may prefer to be called "chemical dependence nurses." In some regions, nurses may work in "rehabilitation programs" and may be referred to as "rehabilitation nurses." Whereas "rehabilitation" may be considered a recovery-oriented approach to addressing problem alcohol and drug use, others may see it as an ambiguous term or may confuse "rehabilitation nurse" as a title for nurses involved in physical and/or injury rehabilitation. In Australasia and Europe, professionals in the addictions nursing specialty are referred to as "alcohol and drug nurses."

In the United States, those in the addictions nursing specialty believe that terms such as "alcohol and drug nurse" are limiting because they exclude other forms of addiction (sometimes referred to as "process addictions" or "behavioral addictions"). These include problem gambling; eating disorders; sex, shopping, internet, or gaming disorders; and other compulsive or harmful behaviors.

STIGMA OF ADDICTION

The classic definition of "stigma" (Goffman, 1963) is a deeply discrediting attribute that reduces someone "from a whole and usual person to a tainted, discounted one" (p. 3) causing that person to be perceived as having a "spoiled identity" (p. 3). Dudley (2000) expanded on Goffman's initial conceptualization to define stigma as "stereotypes or negative views attributed to a person or groups of people when their characteristics or behaviors are viewed as different from or inferior to societal norms" (Ahmedani, 2011, p. 2). Stigmatizing perceptions or judgments occur when one group of individuals labels another group based on preconceived, often false ideas and generalizations. Social prejudices, negative attitudes, and stereotypical perceptions toward individuals with addiction are still common in society and among healthcare professionals (Corrigan et al., 2017). IntNSA has a long-standing role in advocating for individuals, families, communities, and populations affected by the stigma of addiction.

Pejorative, judgmental language about substance use and people who use substances (e.g., terms like "abuse" and "addict") can be stigmatizing (Fraser, 2016). The stigma of addiction can be a barrier to the development of a therapeutic alliance and the initiation or continuation of the individual's recovery process. Addictions nurses advocate for the use of person-first, non-labeling language (e.g., a "person with a substance use disorder" as opposed to an "addict") to minimize the stigma of addiction and promote recovery (Broyles et al., 2014; Burda, 2020; Kelly et al., 2016; Mahmoud et al., 2017). Patients who believe that their healthcare providers have negative attitudes toward them or who perceive that they are being discriminated against can develop mistrust and avoid health care. When internalized, the stigma of addiction, or the fear of it, can become a barrier to treatment, causing individuals to delay or avoid seeking care until their SUD becomes more advanced (Nash et al., 2017).

Additionally, stigmatizing perceptions among nurses and other providers toward patients who use substances may affect their willingness to deliver care for this patient population (Corrigan et al., 2017; Crothers & Dorrian, 2011). To counter the stigma of addiction among nurses and other healthcare professionals, IntNSA recommends incorporating substance use-related content within prelicensure education programs, continuing education offerings, and in-service trainings. Having patients and professional peers who are in recovery as guest speakers may decrease perceptions of stigma and increase empathy (Corrigan et al., 2017; Mahmoud et al., 2018).

CULTURAL COMPETENCE, CULTURAL HUMILITY, AND CULTURALLY CONGRUENT PRACTICE

Culture has been described as

the conceptual system developed by a community or society to structure the way people view the world. It involves a particular set of beliefs, norms, and values that influence ideas about relationships, how people live their lives, and the way people organize their world. (Substance Abuse and Mental Health Services Administration [SAMHSA], 2014a, p. xvi)

Beyond traditional parameters related to race and ethnicity, the word *culture* is sometimes applied to "groups formed on the basis of age, socio-economic status, disability, sexual orientation, [gender orientation], recovery status, common interest, or proximity" (SAMHSA, 2014, p. xvi).

Cultural competence "is a set of congruent behaviors, attitudes, and policies that . . . enable a system, agency, or group of professionals to work effectively in cross-cultural situations" (Cross et al., 1989, p. 13).

As reflected in its position statement, *Cultural and Linguistic Competence*, the International Council of Nurses (ICN, 2013) and its member organizations, which include ANA and IntNSA, believe that nurses should be culturally and linguistically competent to understand and respond effectively to the cultural and linguistic needs of clients, families, and communities in a healthcare encounter. Nurses demonstrate cultural competence by:

- Developing an awareness of one's own culture without letting it have an undue influence on those from other backgrounds,
- Demonstrating knowledge and understanding of different cultures,
- Accepting that there may be differences between cultural beliefs and values of the healthcare provider and the client,
- Accepting and respecting cultural differences,
- Adapting care to be congruent with the client's culture and expectations, and
- Providing culturally appropriate care so as to deliver the best possible client outcomes (ICN, 2013, p. 1).

Cultural humility is distinguishable from cultural competence in that it is "other-oriented" (open to others) rather than self-focused and emphasizes respect and lack of superiority toward another individual's cultural worldview (Hook et al., 2013). Nurses can be experts in many things, but they must engage with patients with an attitude of humility and have a willingness to learn from individuals with different cultural backgrounds. Cultural humility involves having an interest and curiosity about the patient's culture, demonstrating skills in working with diverse cultures, and being willing to engage with patients from other cultures. According to Hook et al. (2013), these attitudes are important aspects of forming strong therapeutic alliances with the patients we serve, and patient perceptions of their healthcare provider's cultural humility are positively associated with positive outcomes of therapy.

In 2015, the American Nurses Association (ANA) published the third edition of *Nursing: Scope and Standards of Practice*, which included, for the first time, a standard for Culturally Competent Practice, "Standard 8: Culturally Congruent Practice: The registered nurse practices in a manner that is congruent with cultural diversity and inclusion principles" (ANA, 2015b, p. 69). The associated practice statement asserted that

> *Culturally congruent practice* is the application of evidence-based nursing that is in agreement with the preferred cultural values, beliefs, worldview, and practices of the healthcare consumer and other stakeholders. Cultural competence represents the process by which nurses demonstrate culturally congruent practice. Nurses design and direct culturally congruent practice and services for diverse consumers to improve access, promote positive outcomes, and reduce disparities. (ANA, 2015b, p. 31)

The Office of Minority Health has issued *National Standards for Culturally and Linguistically Appropriate Services (CLAS) in Health and Health Care*. The principal standard in this document prompts responsible entities to "provide effective, equitable, understandable, and respectful quality care and services that are responsive to diverse cultural beliefs and practices, preferred languages, health literacy, and other communication needs" (Office of Minority Health, 2013, p. 1).

Specific to behavioral health (i.e., mental health, substance use, and related disorders), SAMHSA published *Treatment Improvement Protocol 59: Improving Cultural Competence*. The authors emphasized that

> Counselors and other behavioral health service providers who are equipped with a general understanding of how culture affects their own worldviews as well as those of their clients will be able to work more effectively with clients who have substance use and mental disorders. (SAMHSA, 2014a, pp. 1–2)

Associated attitudes and behaviors of culturally competent clinicians include respect, acceptance, sensitivity, commitment to equality, openness, humility, and flexibility (SAMHSA, 2014a, pp. 49–50). Cultural competence, cultural humility, and culturally congruent practice require nurses to engage in ongoing self-assessment and a lifelong process of professional development (Marion et al., 2017).

Current Issues and Trends in Addictions Nursing

COVID-19 AND SUBSTANCE USE

Individuals who smoke, vape, use opioids, or have a substance use disorder (SUD) are particularly vulnerable for acquiring infectious diseases, including infection with the coronavirus (COVID-19). Risk for severe COVID-19 complications and death is concentrated among those who are immunocompromised, have comorbid conditions, or engage in risky behaviors. People who smoke or inhale substances may already have compromised pulmonary function, due to illnesses like "popcorn lung" (e-cigarette- or vaping-associated lung injury), which can worsen the prognosis and increase the risk of death from COVID-19. Additionally, individuals who use opioids experience respiratory depression and hypoxemia, which can increase the likelihood of death due to both COVID-19 and overdoses (Volkow, 2020).

According to Dr. Nora Volkow, the director of the National Institute on Drug Abuse (NIDA), hospitals that are pushed to (or beyond) their capacity may be inclined to "deprioritize" care for persons with SUD that present with COVID-19 symptoms. It is incumbent on all healthcare workers to treat substance-using individuals with the same compassion and dignity provided to any other patients (Volkow, 2020).

Social isolation and stress are risk factors for relapse. The social isolation that has resulted from infection control efforts during the global COVID-19 pandemic are particularly difficult for individuals with SUDs. Many individuals sustain their recovery efforts via peer support or twelve-step programs. Some individuals with internet access found virtual peer support meetings to be useful, while some felt that virtual meetings were a poor substitute for in-person meetings. Others without internet connectivity have encountered limited access to peer support.

While online meetings are available 24 hours a day, many in recovery have found it difficult to feel engaged.

In general, when people are isolated and stressed, they may turn to substances to alleviate their negative feelings (Volkow, 2020). In a cross-sectional survey of U.S. adults conducted during the pandemic, those who revealed pandemic-related stressors also reported consuming more drinks over a greater number of days, which is concerning from both a clinical and a population public health perspective (Grossman et al., 2020).

Access to quality SUD treatment access was limited even before the COVID-19 pandemic (Guyer & Scott, 2020). Stay at home orders and indoor capacity restrictions have made it even more difficult for individuals to initiate and sustain attendance in treatment and recovery services. Most programs reduced the hours of operation at drop-in centers for needle exchange, supervised injection sites, or other harm reduction services. Other programs simply closed their doors.

Prior to COVID-19, individuals with OUD who received medications like methadone or buprenorphine from federally regulated opioid treatment programs (OTPs) were required to make daily or otherwise routine in-person visits. To ensure accessibility of necessary therapy, in March 2020, the Drug Enforcement Agency (DEA) of the U.S. Department of Justice (DOJ) exercised its authority to provide flexibility in the prescribing of controlled substances. For example, the DEA issued policies for the duration of the public health emergency, which authorized practitioners to prescribe controlled substances to new and existing patients via telemedicine (DOJ DEA, 2020).

In March 2020, SAMHSA issued guidance to enable patients who receive treatment at an OTP to continue to receive medications with longer periods between visits. This allowed states to request blanket exceptions of 14 to 28 days of take-home doses if the OTP deemed that the patient was stable enough to handle this (SAMHSA, 2020b). While these policies helped to maintain access to therapeutic medications during the pandemic, there have been some concerns about potential for diversion and overdose deaths, especially among less stable patients.

LEGALIZATION OF CANNABIS

The International Nurses Society on Addictions' (IntNSA) mission is to "advance excellence in nursing care for the prevention and treatment of addictions"; thus, the Society does not support any use of tobacco, excessive use of alcohol, and the nonprescribed use of psychoactive drugs (including recreational use of cannabis), especially among underage youth, pregnant women, and individuals with, or at risk of developing, psychiatric disorders. As a professional specialty nursing organization, historically IntNSA has not addressed the use of medical cannabis, because cannabis is classified under the Controlled Substances Act as a Schedule I substance with "no accepted medical use" and "a high potential for abuse and the potential to create severe psychological and/or physical dependence" (DOJ DEA, n.d., para. 1). However, a growing number of states have legalized "medical cannabis." It is understood that evidence has emerged regarding the efficacy and accepted use of cannabinoids (i.e., medical cannabis) as a complementary or alternative treatment for a variety of conditions, including seizure disorders, chemotherapy-related nausea and vomiting, AIDS-related weight lost (or "wasting"), intractable pain, and other disorders (National Academies of Sciences, Engineering & Medicine, 2017; Volkow et al., 2014). Therefore, it is important that IntNSA continues to work with pain management and other professional organizations to develop its official position on the use of medical cannabis.

Numerous states have legalized the recreational use of cannabis since 2012, when Colorado became the first state to allow legal sales of nonmedical cannabis for adults over the age of 21. As medical and recreational cannabis becomes more readily accessible, nursing and public health interventions should target the public's awareness of the risks of cannabis. In the 3 years following legalization, Colorado observed a number of consequences pertaining to health behaviors and health outcomes. Poison center call data found a 63% increase in unintentional exposures by infants and children, mostly due to ingestion of "edible" products (e.g., snacks, candies, and other foods infused with cannabinoids). Hospitalizations with cannabis-related codes increased by 70%; emergency department visits increased by 19%; and driving under the influence (DUI) where cannabis was the impairing substance increased by 16% (Ghosh et al., 2017). According to an analysis of National Highway Traffic Safety data, legalization of recreational cannabis is associated with increased traffic fatality rates (Kamer et al., 2020). Also, when smoked, cannabis significantly increases risks of developing respiratory disorders and can affect the body's ability to fight diseases, especially among those who are already immunocompromised (National Academies of Sciences, Engineering & Medicine, 2017; Volkow et al., 2014).

Further, there are significant associations between cannabis and other SUDs, including nicotine dependence, although these associations are influenced by the amount of the substance used, the age at first use, and genetic vulnerability (NIDA, 2020d). According to NIDA, cannabis use is also linked to an increased risk for psychiatric disorders, including psychosis, depression, and anxiety. Compared with those who do not use, those who smoke high-potency cannabis on a daily basis are at nearly five times greater risk of developing psychosis (NIDA, 2020a). Compared with those in early and late adolescence, young adults in states with medical cannabis laws are significantly more likely to have initiated past year cannabis use (Schmidt et al., 2019). According to Schmidt et al. (2019), "Young adults are in the peak years of engagement with illicit drugs and state medical cannabis laws appear to be driving larger numbers to try the drug." Use of cannabis in adolescents and young adults can alter normal development and cognitive functioning, causing neurodevelopmental and neurocognitive effects which can endure into adulthood (Schmidt et al., 2019; Volkow et al., 2014, 2016).

OPIOID CRISIS (THE OPIOID EPIDEMIC)

Opioid use has become a public health crisis with devastating consequences, including increases in overdoses, prenatal opioid use, and criminal violence. Injection and other risky drug use behaviors have also contributed to the spread of infectious diseases (e.g., HIV, hepatitis, endocarditis). These and other medical comorbidities are driving increases in healthcare costs (emergency department and/or hospital utilization). According to NIDA (2020b), roughly 21% to 29% of patients prescribed opioids for chronic pain misuse them, and between 8% and 12% develop a subsequent opioid use disorder. An estimated 4% to 6% who misuse prescription opioids transition to use of heroin or other illicit drugs. About 80% of people who use heroin first misused prescription opioids.

Controlled substance regulation changes, insurance coverage for prescribed opioids, and the use of prescription drug monitoring program (PDMP) databases have reduced the availability of opioids for pain. However, some patients with uncontrolled pain and/or opioid dependence have turned to illicit use of heroin or synthetic opioids such as fentanyl. Thus, while there have been significantly fewer prescriptions written for opioids in the past few years, the unchecked use of opioids and related overdoses have continued to grow. The opioid overdose epidemic was identified as a key contributing factor to decreases in American life expectancy for 2 consecutive years (2015 and 2016), the first 2-year drop in life expectancy since the 1960s (Kochanek et al., 2017; Thielking, 2017).

SOCIAL DETERMINANTS OF HEALTH AND THE EPIDEMIC OF DESPAIR

Addressing the current opioid crisis and other substance use problems involves confronting socioeconomic disparities (NIDA, 2017) in addition to other "demand reduction" efforts. Reducing access to opioids and increasing access to opioid use disorder treatment are critically important, but they are insufficient to address these complex disorders with multiple etiologies. Researchers have documented associations between "social determinants of health" (SDOH) and drug use and drug-related mortality (Blumenthal & Seervai, 2017; Ronka et al., 2017). It is believed that SUDs may be strongly influenced by the "epidemic of despair," a phenomenon first mentioned in 2005. It describes health conditions known to decrease life expectancy, including SUD, that are attributable to SDOH—unemployment, poor finances, lack of education, divorce, depression, loss of social connections, and so forth (Case & Deaton,

2005a, 2005b). "As long as there is distress and despair, some people are going to seek chemical ways to feel better" (Szalavitz, 2016, para. 13). It is important that addictions nurses consider the importance of SDOH (joblessness, poverty) and economic remedies (housing, job training) in addition to addiction rehabilitation services.

SUICIDES AND OPIOID OVERDOSES

While drug overdose deaths have decreased by 4% from 2017 to 2018, the number of drug overdose deaths was still four times higher in 2018 than in 1999. Nearly 70% of all drug overdose deaths involve an opioid, including prescription and illegal opioids such as heroin and illicitly manufactured fentanyl (Centers for Disease Control and Prevention [CDC], 2020d).

Suicides have been identified as a "silent contributor" to high rates of opioid overdose deaths (Oquendo & Volkow, 2018). About 82% of drug overdose deaths in the United States are classified as *unintentional* (accidental), and 12% are classified as *intentionally self-inflicted* (suicide by drug overdose). Suicide rates have increased 30% in nearly every state from 1999 through 2016 (CDC, 2018b), and opioids contribute to 50% of *self-inflicted drug overdose deaths* (Austin et al., 2017). More than half of suicide decedents (54%) were people with no known mental health condition. Since death certificates may not specify whether an overdose involved an opioid or whether it was intentionally self-inflicted (e.g., if there was no suicide note), these data do not accurately capture the true magnitude of the "twin epidemics" of suicide and overdose deaths (Oquendo & Volkow, 2018).

Addictions nurses can anticipate that all patients who use opioids are at increased risk for both accidental and intentional overdose. Suicide completion is strongly correlated with the number and amount of substances used and the severity of substance dependence (Borges et al., 2006; Voss et al., 2013). Screening for suicide intent and providing targeted suicide prevention strategies for those at higher risk due to OUD or chronic pain are important risk mitigation strategies (Voss et al., 2013; Wilcox et al., 2004).

TRAUMA, RESILIENCE, AND TRAUMA-INFORMED CARE

Trauma is defined by exposure to actual or threatened death, serious injury, or sexual violence in one or more ways. According to the 5th edition of the *Diagnostic and Statistical Manual of Mental Disorders* (*DSM-5*), this can include directly experiencing the event, directly witnessing the event occurring to others, learning that such an event happened to a close family member or friend, or experiencing repeated or extreme exposure to aversive details of those events, such as those experienced by first responders as a part of their work (American Psychiatric Association, 2013). These events, series of events, or set of circumstances are experienced by an individual as physically or emotionally harmful or life threatening. Trauma impacts every aspect of the individual's physical health, thoughts, feelings, and beliefs. Responses to such exposures may have lasting adverse effects on an individual's ability to function (SAMHSA, 2014d).

Patients receiving behavioral health services must be assessed for emotional trauma because while many individuals report at least one traumatic event, most, especially those seeking substance use or mental health services, have been exposed to multiple or chronic traumatic events (Ford, 2013; SAMHSA, 2014b). According to the *DSM-5*, to be diagnosed as having traumatic stress or trauma-related disorders, the individual must be assessed for three stages of trauma, including exposure to the precipitating traumatic event, a perception of threat, and a response to that treat (American Psychiatric Association, 2013). Patients may also be diagnosed with criteria that meet other disorders, such as depression, anxiety, or SUD, but these diagnoses will not fully capture the complexity or behaviors.

A "trauma-informed approach" incorporates three key elements: "(1) realizing the prevalence of trauma; (2) recognizing how trauma affects all individuals involved with the program, organization, or system, including its own workforce; and (3) responding by putting this knowledge into practice" (SAMHSA, 2014b, p. 11). Trauma-informed care is an evidence based intervention and organizational approach that focuses on how trauma may have affected an individual and their response to behavioral health services. In a trauma-informed program, policies, procedures, and practices are in place to protect the vulnerabilities of those who have experienced trauma and those who provide trauma-related services. Staff in trauma-informed services are trained and aware of the signs and symptoms of trauma and understand its comprehensive implications.

Harris and Fallot (2001) developed basic principles of trauma-informed care: safety; trustworthiness and transparency; peer support; collaboration and mutuality; empowerment, voice, and choice; and cultural issues. All staff, providers, and environments must prioritize safety in all interactions. Patients must feel safe in order to enhance the second principal of trust and transparency in all treatment plans and decisions. Modeling these concepts may be new to them, and this modeling is a way to enhance personal change in healthy interactions and relationships. Building trust with the organization is foundational to patient participation in program activities and peer support. Supportive interactions help to instill hope and recovery. This purposeful progression allows a deeper experience and understanding of mutuality and collaboration.

The organization allows each individual staff and client alike to empower their voices and make healthy choices through shared decision-making. Lastly the client must acknowledge and address the stigmatizing barriers of culture, gender, and historical trauma. This final process necessitates that the organization makes protocols and procedures that are inclusive and individually responsive. They also have to address how historical trauma can affect multiple generations. Examples of historical trauma include slavery, discrimination, ethnic cleansing, concentration camps, and racialized mass incarceration. The main focus of trauma-informed care is to limit or prevent any policy, procedure, expectation, treatment modality, or response that will retraumatize the client.

Trauma awareness is an essential strategy for preventing retraumatization; it reinforces the need for providers to reevaluate their usual practices. Even the most standard behavioral health practices can be harmful to individuals with prior traumatic experiences if implemented without recognition or consideration of their trauma histories. For example, if a female patient who has been raped is required to attend group therapy in a mostly male group, she may feel unsafe. In this scenario, the patient may likely be susceptible to retraumatization and would benefit from gender-specific services (SAMHSA, 2014b).

Research has documented strong correlations between experienced traumatic stress and neurodevelopmental and immune system responses, as well as development of risky behaviors that are evident in chronic physical and mental health disorders (SAMHSA, 2014b). Prevention is the key to limiting these adverse effects. In 1998, Filetti et al. conducted a study to evaluate the relationship between adverse childhood events (ACEs) and risk behaviors and disease prevalence in adulthood. They identified seven ACE categories, including psychological, physical, or sexual abuse; violence against mother; and living with household members who were substance users, mentally ill or suicidal, or ever imprisoned. They concluded that the seven ACE categories were strongly interrelated and that persons with multiple categories of childhood exposure were likely to have multiple risk factors for numerous leading causes of death in adults. Multiple ACE studies have since confirmed that witnessing or experiencing life-threatening trauma between the ages of 0 to 17 can disrupt healthy brain development, affect social development, and lead to substance misuse and other unhealthy coping behaviors. The CDC (2019a) has made prevention of ACEs a national focus.

Not everyone who experiences trauma suffers chronic adverse effects. These individuals have or develop emotional resilience. Resilience is a protective factor in which a person adapts well in the face of adversity, trauma, and stress. Resilient people not only "bounce back" and heal; sometimes they also experience profound personal growth (American Psychological Association, 2012). Some people reevaluate their values and redefine what is important after a trauma. Resilient responses can include allowing family and community support, using available resources, asking for assistance, finding their sense of purpose, exploring personal priorities, and participating actively in their community.

Special Populations

CO-OCCURRING SUBSTANCE USE AND PSYCHIATRIC DISORDERS

Individuals with SUDs are more likely to have co-occurring psychiatric disorders, and those with psychiatric disorders are more likely to use substances or have SUDs. Patients with co-occurring disorders (CODs) typically have one or more SUDs as well as one or more psychiatric disorders, such as depressive disorders, bipolar I disorder, posttraumatic stress disorder (PTSD), personality disorders (PDs), anxiety disorders, schizophrenia and other psychotic disorders, attention-deficit hyperactivity disorder (ADHD), and eating and feeding disorders. Both disorders are considered primary diagnoses (Minkoff & Covell, 2019). "Co-occurring" or "co-morbidity" does not simply refer to a cluster of symptoms resulting from each type of disorder. Co-morbidity is established when at least one disorder of each type can be identified independently from the other diagnosis and the interactions between both illnesses worsen the course of each disorder (Substance Abuse and Mental Health Services Administration [SAMHSA], 2020a).

People with CODs usually have high levels of problem severity in multiple dimensions, including interpersonal and functional skill deficits, and may require services at a higher acuity level to address their needs. Individuals with CODs may require intensive SUD and mental health treatment, as well as a comprehensive array of additional support services, such as housing, employment, transportation, and case management. Services for people with CODs may be categorized as non-emergency services; emergency services for those in crisis; outreach to target nontreatment seeking individuals and those with great need and/or access barriers; and involuntary, coerced, or mandated services (SAMHSA, 2020a).

Despite high levels of CODs, only 50% of SUD treatment facilities and only 46% of mental health services facilities offer COD-specific programming. Individuals with serious CODs often experience numerous unmet needs, including lack of accurate and timely assessment, diagnostic, and treatment services. The gap between the treatment needed and the services provided may be attributed to a lack of adequate treatment capacity, especially integrated treatment, and provider beliefs that individuals with CODs require more care or a higher level of care than the program can provide. Other barriers to care include healthcare provider shortages, access barriers (e.g., geographic distance, transportation, insurance coverage), and insufficient training in the unique needs of individuals with CODs (SAMHSA, 2020a).

The following six guiding principles can enhance recovery and treatment effectiveness for patients with complex CODs (SAMHSA, 2020a):

1. Use a perspective focused on recovery,
2. Allow for integration of a multiproblem perspective,
3. Plan for a multileveled approach to treatment,
4. Address real-life issues such as childcare and housing early,
5. Identify and adapt the plan of care to the patient's cognitive ability, and
6. Integrate the patient's social supports to their plan of care.

While the six guiding principles are helpful in improving the quality and efficacy of treatment, an ideal treatment delivery system focuses on these six core components (SAMHSA, 2020a):

1. Improving access,
2. Completing comprehensive assessments,
3. Providing appropriate levels of care,
4. Achieving integrated behavioral health treatment,
5. Providing comprehensive treatment services, and
6. Ensuring continuity of care.

Nurses can adapt treatment services to strengthen the patient's resilience, prevent a cascade of negative events, and promote recovery (SAM-

HSA, 2020a). Fundamental provider attitudes include empathy, respect, and belief in the individual's capacity for recovery. The most important predictor of success is the quality of the therapeutic relationship between the patient and provider (Minkoff & Covell, 2019).

CO-OCCURRING SUBSTANCE USE AND CHRONIC PAIN

In 2018, the American Nurses Association (ANA) issued a position statement, *The Ethical Responsibility to Manage Pain and the Suffering it Causes*, to clarify the nurse's role in pain management. All nurses have an ethical imperative to assist their patients to receive appropriate pain management, as well as to consider pain as the patient defines it. In the literature, pain is defined as "an unpleasant sensory and emotional experience associated with, or resembling that associated, actual or potential tissue damage" (International Association for the Study of Pain, 2020, para. 3). Pain is subjective and may not always be corroborated by objective data (SAMHSA, 2012c).

Chronic pain and SUDs frequently co-occur. Both have shared neurophysiological patterns involving abnormal neural processing, may share certain behavioral components, and may have similar physical, social, emotional, and economic effects on health and well-being. Both conditions can be treated effectively with ongoing management and multimodal interventions, yet treatment for one condition may conflict with or support treatment for the other. For example, reliance on prescribed opioid medications for chronic pain may lead to the onset of a SUD, and untreated pain can lead to SUD relapse (SAMHSA, 2012c). While not all patients will develop an addiction with opioid use, any use of opioids puts individuals at risk for development of opioid use disorder (OUD).

Treatment for chronic pain that integrates evidence-based nonpharmacological and pharmacological approaches to ease pain can support maximum quality of life and reduce reliance on medication. Nonpharmacological treatment for chronic pain includes therapeutic exercise, physical therapy, cognitive-behavioral therapy, and complementary and alternative medicine, such as chiropractic treatment, massage therapy, acupuncture, and relaxation training (SAMHSA, 2012c; Thomas, 2020). Pharmacologic treatment for pain includes both nonopioid and opioid medications.

Nonopioid pharmacological management of pain can include prescribed or over-the-counter *analgesics* (acetaminophen); *nonsteroidal anti-inflammatory drugs* (NSAIDs) such as aspirin, ibuprofen, celecoxib, and indomethacin; *anticonvulsant drugs* such as gabapentin; and some *antidepressant medications* (e.g., duloxetine, amitriptyline).

Opioid medications can be quite effective for both acute and chronic pain as a component in an individualized treatment plan. However, the risks of prolonged opioid therapy, which include overdose and OUD, can outweigh the benefits for some patients. Patients with histories of SUD and mental health disorders (MHD) are among the most vulnerable (Brennan, 2020).

While opioids have a place in treatment, opioids alone must not continue to be the go-to solution. Nor should opioid medications be ruled out for individuals with pain based solely on their having a SUD or MHD history. The pain condition and the SUD/MHD can have serious harmful consequences if untreated, and treatment for both comorbidities should be integrated and treated simultaneously (SAMHSA, 2012c).

As the patient's advocate, nurses attend to the patient's overall function and communicate with the interdisciplinary team to adjust the treatment plan as needed. Collaborative advocacy for patients with SUD/MHD, often a highly stigmatized patient population, highlights nurses' ethical imperative. Addictions nurses, pain management nurses, and nurses in all treatment settings must understand and address the needs of patients with persistent pain and SUD/MHD (Fogger & Dobbs, 2020).

NURSES AND NURSING STUDENTS WITH SUBSTANCE USE

The prevalence of SUDs among nurses is similar to that of the general population (Kunyk, 2015). Alcohol and other substance use by nurses potentially place patients, the public, and nurses themselves at risk for serious injury or death (Strobbe & Crowley, 2017). Consequences may include impaired practice, defined as "functioning poorly or with diminished competence, as evident in changes in work habits, job performance, appearance, or other behaviors that may occur in any role or any setting" (ANA, 2015a, p. 43). Some instances involve drug diversion, defined as "the illegal distribution or abuse of prescription drugs or their use for purposes unintended purposes" (Centers for Medicare and Medicaid Services, 2014, p. 3). Nursing students are also at risk for problems related to substance use (ANA, 2015a). Addictions nurses have a long history of advocacy for peer assistance for nurses with impaired practice. Recognizing that treatment works and recovery is possible, nurses in this specialty promote alternative-to-discipline programs (Monroe et al., 2008; Strobbe & Crowley, 2017). "In instances of impaired practice, nurses within all professional relationships must advocate for appropriate assistance, treatment, and access to fair institutional and legal processes. Advocacy includes supporting the return to practice of individuals who have sought assistance" (ANA, 2015a, p. 13). According to Fowler (2015), "Impairment is a matter of compassion and care when the impaired person is a patient. It should be the same when the impaired person is a colleague—or one's self. Intervention is required but it should be compassionate and caring and should seek not only assessment and treatment but where possible, restoration to practice" (p. 53).

The International Nurses Society on Addictions (IntNSA) and the Emergency Nurses Association (ENA) have published a joint position statement, "Substance Use Among Nurses and Nursing Students" (Strobbe & Crowley, 2017). This position statement has been endorsed by ANA, the American Association of Nurse Anesthetists (AANA), the Association of periOperative Registered Nurses (AORN), and the National Organization of Alternative Programs (NOAP). It was widely disseminated by the National Council of State Boards of Nursing (NCSBN).

It is the position of International Nurses Society on Addictions and ENA that

1. Healthcare facilities provide education to all nurses and other employees regarding alcohol and other drug use, and establish

policies, procedures, and practices to promote safe, supportive, drug-free workplaces.

2. Healthcare facilities and schools of nursing adopt alternative-to-discipline (ATD) approaches to treating nurses and nursing students with SUDs, with stated goals of retention, rehabilitation, and reentry into safe, professional practice.

3. Drug diversion, in the context of personal use, is viewed primarily as a symptom of a serious and treatable disease and not exclusively as a crime.

4. Nurses and nursing students are aware of the risks associated with substance use, impaired practice, and drug diversion and have the responsibility and means to report suspected or actual concerns.

When viewed and treated as a chronic medical illness, treatment outcomes for individuals with SUD are comparable to those for other diseases—including asthma, diabetes, and hypertension—and can result in lasting benefits (McLellan et al., 2000). Professional monitoring programs that employ an ATD approach have demonstrated effectiveness in the treatment of health professionals with SUD and are considered a standard for recovery, with high rates of completion and successful return to practice (DuPont et al., 2009; McLellan et al., 2008). In addition, ATD programs have been shown to identify and enroll more nurses with SUDs, with potentially greater impact on protecting the public than disciplinary programs (Monroe et al., 2013).

LESBIAN, GAY, BISEXUAL, TRANSGENDER, QUEER, INTERSEX, AND ASEXUAL (LGBTQIA)

It is important to consider the health needs of nontraditional and marginalized sexual and gender minority groups (SAMHSA, 2012b, 2012d; NIDA, n.d.). This sexual and gender minority category includes individuals (across the lifespan) and families who identify as lesbian, gay, bisexual, transgender, queer, intersex, and asexual (LGBTQIA).

All nurses should be familiar with the following terms, as described here (SAMHSA, 2012d; Amnesty International, n.d.):

- *Lesbian*: A person who self-identifies as female who is attracted romantically, erotically, and/or emotionally to other females.
- *Gay*: A term used in some cultural settings to represent a person who self-identifies as male who has an emotional, sexual, and/or relational attraction to other males.
    - *Note: The term gay may be used by some women who prefer it over the term lesbian.*
    - *Not all men who engage in "same sex behavior" identify as gay, and as such this label should be used with caution.*
    - *Sometimes this term is used to refer to the LGBTQIA community as a whole, or as an individual identity label for anyone who does not identify as heterosexual.*
- *Bisexual*: A person who self-identifies as having an emotional, sexual, and/or relational attraction to men and women.
- *Transgender*: A person whose gender identity and/or expression is different from that typically associated with their assigned sex at birth.
    - *Note: The term transgender has been used to describe a number of gender minorities, including, but not limited to, transsexuals, cross-dressers, androgynous people, genderqueers, and gender nonconforming people.*
    - *"Trans" is shorthand for "transgender."*
- *Queer*: A term usually used to refer to specific sexual orientations (e.g., lesbian, gay, bisexual).
    - *Note: Some individuals use queer as an alternative to gay in an effort to be more inclusive, since the term queer does not convey a sense of gender. However, depending on the user, the term can have either a derogatory or an affirming connotation.*
- *Intersex*: A person whose sex a healthcare provider has a difficult time categorizing as either male or female. A person whose combination of chromosomes, gonads, hormones, internal sex organs, and/or genitals differs from one of the two expected patterns.

- *Asexual*: A person who is not sexually attracted to anyone or does not have a sexual orientation.
- *Cisgender*: A person who feels comfortable with the gender identity and gender expression expectations assigned to them based on their physical sex.

Sexual and gender minority groups face significant health disparities linked to social vulnerabilities like racial and gender stigma, social and internalized stigma, discrimination, bullying, harassment, and victimization. These challenges are not encountered by people who identify in the sexual and gender majority (i.e., heterosexual cisgender groups; Reisner et al., 2017). As a result of these and other stressors, sexual and gender minority groups are at increased risk for SUDs and various mental and behavioral health issues (Semlyen et al., 2016).

Adults in sexual minority groups are more likely to have had past-year SUDs (Medley et al., 2016) and to have reported higher percentages of hazardous drinking behaviors (e.g., binge drinking) compared to heterosexual adults (Ward et al., 2014). Lesbian and bisexual women have higher risks for alcohol use disorders (AUDs) and other SUDs, while gay and bisexual men are at greater risk for illicit drug use. SUDs are highly prevalent among transgender individuals, particularly transgender females and youth, which is directly associated with negative health outcomes, including HIV, Hep C, and other infections; suicidality; and other mental health conditions (Green & Feinstein, 2012; Reisner et al., 2016, 2017). Compared to youth who report only same-sex partners, youth who report having partners of both sexes have significantly higher risk profiles, including histories of drug use, suicide attempts, sexual victimization, and having run away from or been removed from the home (Moon et al., 2007).

A greater understanding of sexual and gender minority groups and their substance use and associated health risks provide an essential beginning to creating a positive healthcare environment that affirms all individuals and families across social, psychological, and medical realms (Reisner et al., 2016). Lack of social and psychological affirmation of sexual and gender identity has been shown to negatively impact healthcare utilization and help-seeking behaviors among sexual and gender minority individuals, including delaying preventive health screenings or avoiding needed medical care when ill or injured (Qureshi et al., 2018).

Sexual and gender identity affirming health care is culturally and contextually appropriate, engaging, and affirming to individuals and families in sexual and gender minority groups (Reisner et al., 2016). It is important to engage and support the entire family when caring for this population, as they can become a supportive resource in the recovery process. Recovery from SUD and co-occurring mental health conditions are greatly improved when providers adopt a family and community systems approach to engage and support the family in the recovery process (SAMHSA, 2014c).

Addictions nurses and other health professionals must create safe places for sexual and gender minority groups across all racial and ethnic backgrounds to receive comprehensive SUD treatment. Engagement and retention strategies need to include plans to acknowledge and decrease their vulnerability, particularly stigma, trauma, and discrimination within treatment settings. Decreasing stigma and discrimination can be accomplished by using gender and sexual identity affirming language on office forms and providing continuing education about sexual orientation, cultural congruence, and gender affirmation for healthcare workers and staff (SAMHSA, 2014c). Addictions nurses must equip themselves with greater knowledge on sexual identity, gender affirmation, and health issues that impact these groups. Addictions nurses and other healthcare providers must proactively screen for SUD and co-occurring mental health and physical conditions and educate individuals and their families about their heightened health risks. Nonjudgmental, nonstigmatizing nursing care will promote stronger therapeutic partnerships and lead to positive recovery outcomes for the entire family (SAMHSA, 2014c).

Advocacy and Health Policy in Addictions Nursing

THE TREATMENT GAP, HEALTHCARE REFORM, AND INSURANCE PARITY

The term "treatment gap" commonly refers to a phenomenon wherein individuals are classified as needing but not receiving SUD treatment. In 2015, about 21.7 million people, or 8.1% of individuals aged 12 or older, were classified as needing SUD treatment in the past year, but more than 19 million (89%) of those did not receive treatment (Park-Lee et al., 2017). A lack of health insurance coverage or an inability to afford the cost of treatment has been reported by 27% of those who do not receive the SUD treatment services that they needed (Park-Lee et al., 2017). It is widely accepted that the Patient Protection and Affordable Care Act of 2010 (ACA) has improved healthcare access, quality, and outcomes for individuals with SUDs, yet the ACA remains under threat of repeal (Abraham et al., 2017; American Nurses Association, 2017; Fornili, 2017; Kaiser Family Foundation, 2017; National Council for Behavioral Health, 2017; Office of the Assistant Secretary for Planning and Evaluation, 2016, 2017; Vestal, 2017).

Medicaid expansion is perhaps the most important healthcare reform under the ACA; it is the single largest source of care for people with behavioral health disorders (Orgera & Tolbert, 2019; Zur & Henry, 2017). Medicaid-eligible individuals with SUDs have greater need for higher complexity treatment services because of high rates of medical and psychiatric comorbidity and increased problem severity (Bailey, 2017). Nearly 30% of patients with insurance coverage through Medicaid expansion have SUDs and/or comorbid mental illnesses (Buck, 2011; Dey et al., 2016;

J. Miller, 2013; Paradise, 2017; Toledo, 2017). However, access to behavioral health care remains limited because, as of 2020, only 37 states (including the District of Columbia) have expanded their Medicaid coverage (Kaiser Family Foundation, 2020).

Several states, especially those with the highest opioid overdose death rates, utilize Medicaid to expand access to buprenorphine, naltrexone, and naloxone. In some states, Medicaid pays for 35%–50% of all treatment services that utilize medications (Toledo, 2017). Nationally, Medicaid expansion has reduced unmet need for treatment by over 18% (Bailey, 2017; Office of the Assistant Secretary for Planning and Evaluation, 2017).

The Paul Wellstone and Pete Domenici Mental Health Parity and Addiction Equity Act of 2008 (the "Parity Act") required that plans cover behavioral health services at the same level as health plans for physical conditions. It required that all plans in individual and small-group markets provide certain "essential health benefits" (EHBs). Prescription drug coverage (including medications for SUD treatment) and behavioral health (mental health and SUD) services were included on an approved list of 10 EHBs (Centers for Medicare and Medicaid Services [CMS], n.d.) The Parity Act, combined with the ACA, expanded behavioral health treatment access for people with Medicaid, marketplace, and employer-based insurance (Fornili, 2017).

There are relentless, often politicized threats to repeal the ACA and make tremendous cuts to Medicaid and other social services. This is despite years of improvements realized since the ACA took effect, mostly related to Medicaid expansion efforts to assist low-income, nonelderly adults. Addictions nurses should be alerted to the serious, often lethal consequences that individuals with SUDs will experience if the ACA is repealed or if Medicaid experiences deeper cuts (Fornili, 2017).

BUPRENORPHINE AND PRESCRIPTIVE AUTHORITY FOR ADVANCED PRACTICE REGISTERED NURSES

Numerous federal statutes, regulations, and guidelines govern medications for opioid use disorder (MOUD), specifically, methadone and certain buprenorphine products. The Substance Abuse and Mental Health Services Administration Center for Substance Abuse Treatment Division of Pharmacologic Therapies (SAMHSA-CSAT-DPT) manages day-to-day oversight activities regarding these regulations.

Some medications used in the treatment of opioid use disorders (OUD) are controlled substances governed by the Controlled Substances Act (CSA). The CSA contains federal drug policy for regulating the manufacture, importation, possession, use, and distribution of controlled substances.

The Drug Addiction Treatment Act of 2000 (DATA 2000), part of the Children's Health Act of 2000, permitted only physicians who met certain qualifications to treat opioid dependence with narcotic medications approved by the Food and Drug Administration (FDA)—including buprenorphine—in treatment settings other than regulated opioid treatment programs (OTPs), for example, in office-based opioid treatment (OBOT). DATA 2000 permitted qualified physicians to obtain a waiver from the separate registration requirements of the Narcotic Addict Treatment Act of 1974 to treat opioid dependence with scheduled medications with FDA approval for that indication. This act did not include advanced practice registered nurses as providers.

The Comprehensive Addiction and Recovery Act of 2016 (CARA) was signed into law in 2016 for a comprehensive, coordinated response to the opioid epidemic. It endorsed the use of medications for OUD, and it authorized nurse practitioners (NPs) and physician assistants (PAs) to be granted, for a 5-year period, a waiver to prescribe buprenorphine in accordance with state scope of practice laws, following completion of mandatory training on substance use. The CARA Act also required that, if the state's scope of practice laws required the NP to have a supervisory or collaborative relationship with a physician, the physician also had to be waivered to prescribe buprenorphine. Another provision in CARA made the opioid agonist naloxone more widely available, especially by first responders, for reversal of opioid overdose, in order to save lives (Community Anti-Drug Coalitions of America, n.d.).

The Substance Use Disorder Prevention That Promotes Opioid Recovery and Treatment for Patients and Communities or SUPPORT for

Patients and Communities Act of 2018 (SUPPORT Act) granted permanent authority for NPs and PAs to prescribe buprenorphine for OUD. It also expanded the prescribing of medications for OUD to additional practitioners in various settings, by defining "qualified practitioners" as physicians, NPs, PAs, clinical nurse specialists (CNSs), certified registered nurse anesthetists (CRNAs), and certified nurse-midwives (CNMs).

RACIALIZED MASS INCARCERATION AND THE WAR ON DRUGS

With the massive cost in terms of money and human lives lost to the opioid epidemic, more attention is being directed at the relationships among crime, incarceration, and enforcement of laws related to getting, having, and using drugs (NIDA, 2020c). The United States leads the world in incarceration, having over two million people behind bars. Two thirds of these are people of color (Mauer, 2011).

The War on Drugs is a major contributor to mass incarceration, along with other social and criminal justice policies. Punitive sentencing policies include three-strike and mandatory sentencing laws. Another contributor to mass incarceration is the deinstitutionalization of people with mental illnesses (Davis, 2017; Dyer, 2000; Bobo & Thompson, 2010; Wildeman & Wang, 2017).

Mass incarceration refers to extreme levels of incarceration that are so heavily concentrated among certain groups that it achieves some level of normalcy (Dyer, 2000; Garland, 2001; Wildeman & Wang, 2017). When mass incarceration involves racial profiling, disproportionate use of force, and disparities in arrests, it becomes racialized mass incarceration (Fornili, 2018).

Massive increases in incarceration are the result of a combination of social and criminal justice policies, like the War on Drugs and its "get tough" policies (Mauer, 2011). While there are radically disproportionate racial differences in rates of drug-related arrests, there is no evidence that rates of drug use and distribution vary significantly by race. Only 14% of regular drug users are Black, compared with 26% who are White. However, drug users that are Black constitute almost 34% of drug-related arrests and almost half of drug-related convictions and state prison sentences (Bobo & Thompson, 2010).

Incarceration does little to address SUD, as addictions treatment is rarely available during incarceration. When individuals who are in behavioral health treatment become incarcerated, their treatment may be inadequate, insufficient, unavailable, or prematurely terminated. When individuals with SUD are under- or untreated during incarceration, upon release, their rates of relapse and overdose are very high (Fox et al., 2015; Winkelman et al., 2018).

Studies have found that SUD treatment and social interventions for at-risk families, like preschool programs and incentives for high school completion are more effective and cost-effective than continued prison expansion (Mauer, 2011). Mass incarceration was supposed to control crime, but it has only had a minimal impact on crime rates and is associated with perpetuation and exacerbation of racial inequality. Mass incarceration does not save taxpayers' money, decrease crime, or rehabilitate prisoners (Dyer, 2000; Green, 2006); instead, it compromises the health of involved individuals, their families, and their communities before, during, and after incarceration.

Addictions nurses object to the conditions that perpetuate the War on Drugs and racialized mass incarceration. They have an ethical responsibility to advocate for social justice and healthy sociopolitical environments for all members of society, regardless of race, class, or creed (Fornili, 2018). The War on Drugs has become a war on our own people, particularly people of color, their families, and their communities. Those with criminal justice histories may not qualify for certain types of employment, professional licenses, enlistment in the military, or security clearances. Thus, it is difficult for individuals with SUD who have been incarcerated to fully integrate into society (Fornili, 2018).

Cross-agency coordination and collaboration is effective and will benefit the health, safety, and welfare of all. Recovery efforts can be optimized by investing in social services, community-based alternatives in lieu of incarceration, treatment offered during incarceration with community-based aftercare treatment, drug courts that blend judicial monitoring with sanctions, and treatment coordinated with parole or probation supervision (Sawyer & Wagner, 2019; NIDA, 2014).

RIGHTS UNDER LAWS THAT PROTECT AGAINST DISCRIMINATION

Federal laws prohibit discrimination against "individuals with disabilities," yet individuals in treatment for SUD often face discrimination. This may be due to lack of knowledge about these laws and the value, effectiveness, and safety of treatment. Further, individuals in treatment for SUD may not have the tools necessary to educate employers, landlords, courts, and others about relevant legal protections (Legal Action Center [LAC], 2009).

People in recovery from SUD—including those receiving medications—generally are protected from discrimination by the Americans with Disabilities Act (ADA), the Rehabilitation Act of 1973, the Fair Housing Act (FHA), and the Workforce Investment Act (WIA). Many states and cities also have nondiscrimination laws that protect individuals with disabilities—including those with SUD. This information is available from state and city enforcement agencies.

Under these federal laws, an individual with a "disability" is someone who has a current "physical or mental impairment" that "substantially limits" one or more "major life activities." They must also have records of substantially limiting impairment or be regarded as having such an impairment (LAC, 2009). SUDs can be considered impairments and, for many people, can substantially limit major life activities (e.g., caring for one's self, working). For this reason, many courts have found that people in treatment for SUD have a record of impairment, including those who are undergoing treatment with methadone, buprenorphine, and other MOUD (LAC, 2009).

Health Care

People who *currently* engage in the *illegal* use of drugs are generally not protected under federal nondiscrimination laws, for example, employees who are fired for using cocaine. However, it is important to note that anti-discrimination laws *do* protect individuals with illicit drug use from discrimination by healthcare providers. It is illegal for a healthcare provider to deny medical care, surgery, dental care, and so forth just because the individual uses an illegal drug. Also, healthcare providers are "public accommodations" under the ADA and may not refuse to provide health services to individuals solely because they participate in pharmacologic therapy for SUD treatment (LAC, 2009). Refusal of care for illicit drug use or for participation in SUD treatment is also considered a breach of ethical conduct for nurses and other healthcare providers.

Child Welfare

Individuals being treated for SUD with medications may not be treated less favorably than other individuals simply because they are receiving pharmacological therapies. Judges, prosecuting attorneys, and others in the child welfare system may not require parents to stop treatment in order to get their children back or to keep their children. They cannot be required to stop taking *legally prescribed* medications. Such a requirement would be like telling an insulin-dependent, diabetic parent that they may not have their children back unless they stop taking insulin and address their diabetes through nutrition and exercise alone. Courts may, however, require people receiving pharmacological treatment to comply with SUD treatment requirements (LAC, 2009).

Driving

A department of motor vehicles (DMV) is prohibited under federal anti-discrimination laws from withholding licensure reinstatement based on an individual's participation in SUD treatment. The DMV also may not require individuals charged with "driving under the influence" (DUI) to attend a SUD treatment program that does not use medications like buprenorphine or methadone. However, regulations implemented by the Federal Highway Administration of the U.S. Department of Transportation (DOT) disqualify individuals from receiving an *interstate* commercial driver's license (CDL) if they are taking methadone. Consequently, it is not illegal for the DOT to deny a CDL because of participation in a methadone program, but DOT regulations are silent about treatment with buprenorphine. CDLs for *intrastate* (within one state) driving are determined by state laws (LAC, 2009).

FEDERAL LAWS THAT PROTECT CONFIDENTIALITY AND PRIVACY

Stemming from legislation in the early 1970s, confidentiality when working with patients with substance use is governed by federal law (Confidentiality of Records, 2010) and regulations (Confidentiality of Substance Use Disorder Patient Records, 2017). Thus, long before the Health Insurance Portability and Accountability Act of 1996 (HIPAA), addictions nurses were well informed in the practice of strict confidentiality of information about all persons receiving treatment for substance use. The law and regulations known as "42 CFR Part 2" are designed to protect privacy rights and decrease barriers to treatment that result from the stigmas associated with substance use. Federal confidentiality laws are predicated on the public health view that persons with SUDs are more likely to seek (and succeed at) treatment if they are assured that their need for treatment will not be disclosed unnecessarily to others. 42 CFR Part 2 is intended to ensure that knowledge of one's participation in treatment for SUDs does not result in adverse consequences (e.g., criminal offenses) and domestic proceedings (e.g., child custody, divorce, employment; SAMHSA, n.d.-b).

In keeping with that view, drug and alcohol confidentiality regulations restrict both the disclosure and use of information about individuals in federally assisted drug or alcohol treatment programs (42 C.F.R. § 2.3-a). Federal regulations restrict the disclosure and use of "patient-identifying" information about individuals in treatment for substance use, whether a person is receiving, has received, or has applied for treatment for substance use (42 C.F.R. § 2.11). The regulations apply to holders, recipients, and seekers of patient-identifying information. An individual or program in possession of such information may not release or rerelease it except as authorized by the patient concerned or as otherwise permitted by the regulations (42 C.F.R. § 2.13-b).

Code of Ethics and Addictions Nursing

Ethical concerns in addictions nursing practice are often complex and multidimensional and may or may not be addressed in laws and professional ethics codes (Corey et al., 2018). Codes of ethical practice educate and inform professionals about sound ethical behavior, while mandating a minimal standard of practice. *Code of Ethics for Nurses With Interpretive Statements* (American Nurses Association [ANA], 2015a) is nonnegotiable in any setting and may only be revised or updated by formal procedures established by the ANA. The Code provides a framework for ethical nursing practice in addictions and is a guide for nurses to use in ethical analysis and decision-making. Specific examples of how the Code of Ethics provisions guide addictions nursing practice follow.

PROVISION 1: COMPASSION AND RESPECT

The nurse practices with compassion and respect for the inherent dignity, worth, and unique attributes of every person.

Compassion is a key value of IntNSA and addictions nursing. Compassion means that addictions nurses recognize the importance of helping others through caring. Compassion entails the installation of hope in those who feel hopeless and the empowerment of those who are powerless as a result of substance use disorders and other addictive behaviors. Respect is another key value of nurses caring for individuals and families. Addictions nurses respect the dignity and worth of every individual, based on the understanding that substance use and addictive disorders, like other chronic health problems, have periods of acute illness and remission. Hence, addictions nurses are staunch patient advocates in helping to overcome negative attitudes and beliefs related to addictions to ensure individualized, appropriate, compassionate, and respectful care.

PROVISION 2: PRIMARY COMMITMENT TO THE PATIENT

The nurse's primary commitment is to the patient, whether an individual, family, group, community, or population.

Addictions nurses recognize that substance use and maladaptive behaviors affect the individual, the family and other groups, and society as a whole. There is a progressive sequence of events, although the pace and intensity of the consequences vary from individual to individual. Grounded in neuroscience of addiction, addictions nurses appreciate that substance use is a brain-based disorder, wherein loss of control, compulsive use, continued use despite consequences, and cravings for the substance are hallmarks of the disease process. Addictions nurses also understand behavior change processes, and recognize that, as in any chronic illness, setbacks may occur as the individual moves toward the initiation and maintenance of behavior change in a process of recovery.

Relapse, or reversion to the target behavior, is best conceptualized as a dynamic, ongoing process rather than a discrete or terminal event (Hendershot et al., 2011; White, 2008). With this understanding, addictions nurses do not take a punitive stance toward those who return to the use of alcohol or other drugs, or who return to behavior that is maladaptive (i.e., relapse). Because they understand the pathophysiology of craving, tolerance, and withdrawal, addictions nurses are keen to identify individuals who may be at high risk for relapse. They promote safe environments where associated harms are reduced. To support risk reduction and promote abstinence or harm reduction, addictions nurses actively engage in relapse prevention skills with individuals affected by addictions, as well as their families and other groups.

PROVISION 3: ADVOCACY AND PROTECTION

The addictions nurse promotes, advocates for, and protects the rights, health, and safety of the patient.

Like all nurses, addictions nurses are fundamentally responsible for promoting health, preventing illness, restoring health, and alleviating suffering. Inherent in addictions nursing is "a respect for human rights, including cultural rights, the right to life and choice, to dignity and to be treated with respect. . . . Nursing care is respectful of and unrestricted by considerations of age, colour, creed, culture, disability or illness, gender, sexual orientation, nationality, politics, race or social status" (International Council of Nurses [ICN], 2012, p. 1). Addictions nurses, in providing care, ensure that care is compatible with the safety, dignity, and rights of people and take appropriate actions to safeguard individuals, families, and communities when their health is endangered by coworkers or any other person (ICN, 2012).

PROVISION 4: OBLIGATION TO PROMOTE HEALTH

The addictions nurse has authority, accountability, and responsibility for nursing practice; makes decisions; and takes action consistent with the obligation to promote health and to provide optimal care.

Addictions nurses bear primary responsibility for the care their patients and clients receive and are accountable for their own practice. To be accountable, nurses follow a code of ethical conduct that includes principles such as fidelity, loyalty, veracity, beneficence, and respect for the dignity, worth, and self-determination of patients, as well as adhering to the scope and standards of nursing practice. Addictions nurses are also responsible for assessing their own competence. When their skill level does not match patient care needs, addictions nurses are responsible for seeking consultation or supervision from other nurses or healthcare professionals to ensure the patient receives the best care possible.

Addictions nurses must not engage in practices prohibited by law or delegate activities to others that are prohibited by their state nurse practice acts or the practice acts of other healthcare providers. In every role, addictions nurses have vested authority and are accountable and responsible for the quality of their practice. Addictions nurses must always comply with and adhere to state nurse practice acts, regulations, standards of care, and the ANA *Code of Ethics for Nurses with Interpretive Statements.*

Some states have received complaints about licensed practical/licensed vocational nurse (LPN/LVN) and registered nurse (RN) practices in a number of opioid treatment programs (OTPs). There is concern that medical directors, program physicians, administrators, and supervisors may not fully understand the legal scope of nursing practice. As a result, LPN/LVN have been asked to accept assignments that exceed their scope of practice. However, the legally defined scope of practice cannot be expanded by an employer, a physician, or any other professional in any practice setting. Licensed addictions nurses (RN, LPN/LVN) are responsible and accountable for practicing within their appropriate scope of practice. LPN/LVN practice is dependent and directed at all times; they may participate in assessment and planning but cannot independently perform these activities. Any nurse who accepts assignments that exceed their legally defined scope of practice is not fulfilling their code of ethics and patient care and professional responsibilities (North Carolina Board of Nursing & the North Carolina State Opioid Treatment Authority, 2014).

PROVISION 5: DUTIES TO SELF AND OTHERS

The nurse owes the same duties to self as to others, including the responsibility to promote health and safety, preserve wholeness of character and integrity, maintain competence, and continue personal and professional growth.

Moral respect accords moral worth and dignity to all human beings, regardless of their personal attributes or life situation. When addictions nurses care for those whose health conditions, attributes, lifestyles, or situations are stigmatized, or encounter a conflict with their own personal beliefs, they must render compassionate, respectful, and competent care. Addictions nurses must always make decisions and take actions that are consistent with nursing ideals, values, and the *Code of Ethics for Nurses with Interpretive Statements.* When decisions or actions are morally objectionable, whether intrinsically so or because they may jeopardize the patient, family, community, population, or nursing practice, addictions nurses must communicate conscience-based objections and actively promote alternatives which do not violate the nurse's moral standards.

Respect for others extends to respect for oneself as well. The same duties we owe to others, we owe to ourselves. Addictions nurses model the same health maintenance and health promotion measures that they teach and research, obtain health care when needed, and avoid taking unnecessary risks to health or safety in their professional or personal activities. Fatigue and compassion fatigue affect a nurse's professional performance and personal life. To mitigate these effects, nurses should eat a healthy diet, exercise, get sufficient rest, maintain personal and professional relationships, engage in adequate leisure and recreational activities, avoid use of substances or excessive use of alcohol, and attend to spiritual or religious needs.

Addictions-related stigma is counterproductive and interferes with the recovery process. Addictions nurses are in key roles to change negative attitudes and convey the critical importance of nursing's role in prevention, intervention, treatment, and recovery for individuals impacted by addictive disorders.

PROVISION 6: ETHICAL ENVIRONMENT OF WORK AND ENGAGEMENT

The nurse, through individual and collective effort, establishes, maintains, and improves the ethical environment of the work setting and conditions of employment that are conducive to safe, quality health care.

The workplace must be a moral milieu that ensures ongoing safe, quality patient care and professional satisfaction for nurses and that minimizes and addresses moral distress, strain, and dissonance.

Alcohol and other substance use by nurses and nursing students affects their physiological and psychological fitness. It impedes their ability to perform assigned duties, violates public trust, and places patients, the public, and nurses themselves at risk for serious injury or death.

Addictions nurses are often the first to recognize substance use and addictive behaviors and are instrumental in establishing nonpunitive programs for nurses and other health professionals with drug or alcohol problems. Rather than viewing substance use as a personal weakness characterized by lack of willpower or volitional control, substance-related problems among nurses is a chronic medical illness in need of treatment and professional monitoring.

Position statements, such as "Substance Use Among Nurses and Nursing Students: A Joint Position Statement of the Emergency Nurses Association and the International Nurses Society on Addictions" (Strobbe & Crowley, 2017) outline "alternative-to-discipline" (ATD) approaches, usually administered by a third party through contractual agreements with a state board of nursing. Nurses involved in ATD programs refrain from work while undergoing treatment, are closely monitored, and may experience gradual lifting of restrictions as they demonstrate progress toward meeting their sobriety and recovery goals.

PROVISION 7: ADVANCEMENT OF THE PROFESSION

The nurse, in all roles and settings, advances the profession through research and scholarly inquiry, professional standards development, and the generation of both nursing and health policy.

Addictions nurses participate in the advancement of the profession through knowledge development, evaluation, dissemination, and application to practice. Knowledge development relies chiefly, although not exclusively, upon research and scholarly inquiry. Researchers in addictions nursing draw from and contribute to the science of addiction and recovery. They engage in scholarly inquiry with interdisciplinary colleagues to expand the body of knowledge that forms and advances the theory and practice of the discipline.

Implementation of research findings to practice remains a major concern in the prevention and treatment of substance use and related disorders. For example, screening, brief intervention, and referral to treatment (SBIRT) is an evidence-based practice that can be implemented in any healthcare setting. The purpose of SBIRT is to identify, reduce, and prevent problematic use, misuse, and dependence on alcohol and other drugs, especially at early stages of disease. However, despite more than 50 years of research evidence, screening and brief intervention remain under implemented in many healthcare settings for a variety of reasons (Fornili, 2016a; Rahm et al., 2015; Saitz, 2007). It is the ethical obligation of the nurse to translate science and support evidence-informed nursing practice.

PROVISION 8: COLLABORATION WITH OTHER PROFESSIONALS AND THE PUBLIC

The nurse collaborates with other health professionals and the public to protect human rights, promote health diplomacy, and reduce health disparities.

Addictions nurses believe that health and recovery are universal human rights. This is consistent with views held by ANA, ICN, the United Nations, the World Health Organization, and many human rights treaties. Addictions nurses understand that health as a universal human right has economic, political, social, and cultural dimensions. Achieving and sustaining health is a means to the common good. Addictions nurses commit to advancing health, welfare, safety, and recovery to help individuals live to their fullest potential with dignity. Addictions nurses work within the community to provide consultation and care for individuals across the lifespan within a full-service continuum. Addictions nurses work in collaboration with other health professionals and policymakers to sustain health and promote social justice through ethical practice and protection of human rights. Addictions nurses engage in partnerships with other specialty nurses (e.g., psychiatric mental health, pain management, emergency, surgical, and neonatal nursing), government agencies (e.g., SAMHSA), and others to educate the community about addictive disorders and promote the societal benefits of prevention, treatment, and recovery.

PROVISION 9: INTEGRITY OF THE PROFESSION, SOCIAL JUSTICE, AND POLICY

The profession of nursing, collectively through its professional organizations, must articulate nursing values, maintain the integrity of the profession, and integrate principles of social justice into nursing and health policy.

Health and access to health care are universal human rights. All nurses commit to advancing health, welfare, and safety. Addictions nurses view recovery as a fundamental aspect of health and wellness. They respect the human rights, values, customs, dignity, and spiritual beliefs of individuals, families, and communities. It is the shared responsibility of nurses and professional nursing organizations to advocate collectively to improve health care and levels of wellness. Addictions nurses understand that social determinants of health, including inequality, poverty, and social marginalization, contribute to addictive disorders in particular and deterioration of global health in general. Addictions nurses address health in all contexts and lead collaborative partnerships to develop effective health legislation, policies, and programs to promote and restore health, prevent illness, and alleviate suffering. For example, addictions nurses advocate for policy changes that improve access to nonpunitive substance use treatment for women who are pregnant and those who want to breastfeed, as well as the vulnerable children who have been exposed to substances.

Standards of Addictions Nursing Practice

SIGNIFICANCE OF THE STANDARDS

The Standards of Professional Nursing Practice are authoritative statements of the duties that all registered nurses, regardless of role, population, or specialty, are expected to perform competently. The standards published herein may serve as evidence of the standard of care, with the understanding that application of the standards is context dependent. The standards are subject to change with the dynamics of the nursing profession, as new patterns of professional practice are developed and accepted by the nursing profession and the public. In addition, specific conditions and clinical circumstances may also affect the application of the standards at a given time (e.g., during a natural disaster). The standards are subject to formal, periodic review and revision.

Healthcare consumer refers to "the patients, persons, clients, families, groups, communities, or populations who are the focus of attention and to whom the registered nurse is providing services as sanctioned by the state regulatory bodies. This more global term is intended to reflect a proactive focus on health and wellness care, rather than a reactive perspective to disease and illness" (American Nurses Association [ANA], 2015b, p. 2).

ADDICTIONS NURSING COMPETENCIES

The competencies that accompany each of the following standards provide evidence of compliance with the corresponding standard. The list of competencies is not exhaustive. Whether a standard or competency applies to a particular situation depends upon the circumstances. The competencies are presented for the registered nurse level and are applicable for *all* nurses. Standards may include additional competencies delineated for the graduate-level prepared registered nurse, a category that also includes advanced practice registered nurses. In some instances, additional discrete competencies applicable only to advanced practice registered nurses may be included. The competencies within the *Addictions Nursing: Scope and Standards of Practice* are designed to promote assessment of the addictions nurse's performance and ongoing attainment of competencies required for safe and responsible practice (American Association of Colleges of Nursing, 2021).

THE NURSING PROCESS AND STANDARDS OF PROFESSIONAL NURSING PRACTICE MODEL

Nurses as scientists rely on qualitative and quantitative evidence to guide policies and practices but also as a way of identifying the nurse's impact on the patient's health outcomes. When describing how nurses critically think and perform professional activities, the nursing process emerges as a commonly used analytical framework.

The *nursing process critical thinking model* supports evidence-based practice and is conceptualized as a cyclic, iterative, and dynamic process that includes assessment, diagnosis, outcomes identification, planning, implementation, and evaluation.

The Standards of Practice (Standards 1–6) are represented in the first ring of the "Nursing Process and Standards of Professional Nursing Practice" model (Figure 3). These standards describe a *competent level of nursing practice* that corresponds to the steps of the nursing process.

The Standards of Professional Performance (Standards 7–17) are identified in the outer ring of the model. These describe a *competent level of behavior in the professional role* appropriate to the nurse's education and position and reflect how the professional nurse adheres to the Standards of Practice, completes the nursing process, and addresses other nursing practice issues and concerns.

The public has a right to expect registered nurses specializing in substance use and addictive disorders to demonstrate addictions nursing

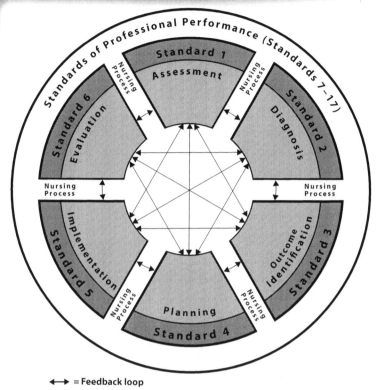

← → = Feedback loop

From: *Nursing Scope and Standards of Practice* (3rd ed., p. 14), American
Nurses Association, 2015.

competence (i.e., performing at an expected level) throughout their
careers. The addictions nurse is individually responsible and accountable
for maintaining professional competence. The nursing profession and
regulatory agencies define minimal standards of competence to protect
the public. The employer is responsible and accountable to provide a
practice environment conducive to competent practice. Assurance of
competence is the shared responsibility of the profession, individual
addictions nurses, professional organizations, credentialing and certification entities, regulatory agencies, employers, and other key stakeholders (ANA, 2014).

Standards of Practice for Addictions Nursing

STANDARD 1. ASSESSMENT

The addictions registered nurse collects pertinent data and information relative to the healthcare consumer's health and/or the situation.

Competencies

The addictions registered nurse:

- Collects pertinent data, including but not limited to demographics; social determinants of health; health disparities; and physical, functional, psychosocial, emotional, cognitive, sexual, cultural, age-related, environmental, spiritual, transpersonal, and economic assessments in a systematic, ongoing process with compassion and respect for the inherent dignity, worth, and unique attributes of every person.
- Assesses for psychoactive substance toxicity, intoxication, and withdrawal symptoms; aggression or danger to others; potential for self-inflicted harm or suicide; and co-occurring mental disorders.
- Collects information on the amount, frequency, and pattern of alcohol, tobacco, and/or drug (ATOD) use; comorbid conditions; and behaviors that may be maladaptive.
- Systematically gathers data from the healthcare consumer and other available collateral sources (family, other healthcare providers) as appropriate in holistic data collection, using screening instruments and other methods that are sensitive to age, developmental level, culture, and gender. At a minimum, data should include current and historic substance use; health, mental health, and substance-related treatment histories; mental

and functional statuses; and current social, environmental, and/or economic constraints.

- Recognizes the importance of the assessment parameters identified by the World Health Organization (WHO), *Healthy People 2030*, the International Nurses Society on Addictions (IntNSA), and other organizations that influence addictions nursing practice.
- Recognizes that crisis may indicate an underlying substance use disorder and may be a window of opportunity for change.
- Assists the patient in identifying the effect of substance use on their current life problems and the effects of continued harmful use.
- Determines the patient's level of readiness to change their substance use behaviors and enter treatment if indicated.
- Elicits the healthcare consumer's values, preferences, expressed and unexpressed needs, and knowledge of the healthcare situation, especially related to prevention and treatment of substance use, addictive disorders, and the process of recovery.
- Recognizes the impact of one's own personal attitudes, values, and beliefs on the assessment process.
- Identifies barriers to effective communication based on psychosocial, literacy, financial, and cultural considerations.
- Assesses impact of family dynamics on healthcare consumer health and wellness.
- Prioritizes data collection based on the healthcare consumer's immediate condition or anticipated needs.
- Utilizes evidence-based screening and assessment instruments to identify patterns and variances in available information, such as the Alcohol Use Disorders Identification Test (AUDIT); Drug Abuse Screening Test (DAST); Alcohol, Smoking, Substance Involvement Screening Test (ASSIST); or the National Institute on Drug Abuse (NIDA) single screening question for drug use: "How many times in the past year have you used an illegal drug or used a prescription medication for nonmedical reasons?" (Smith et al., 2010).

- Applies ethical, legal, and privacy guidelines and policies to the collection, maintenance, use, and dissemination of data and information.
- Recognizes healthcare consumers as the authority on their own health by honoring their care preferences.
- Documents relevant data accurately and in a manner accessible to the interprofessional team.

ADDITIONAL COMPETENCIES FOR THE GRADUATE-LEVEL PREPARED REGISTERED NURSE IN THE ADDICTIONS SPECIALTY

In addition to the competencies of the addictions registered nurse, the graduate-level prepared addictions registered nurse:

- Assesses the effect of interactions among individuals, family, community, and social systems on health and illness.
- Synthesizes the results and information to clinical understanding.

ADDITIONAL COMPETENCIES FOR THE ADVANCED PRACTICE REGISTERED NURSE IN THE ADDICTIONS SPECIALTY

In addition to the competencies of the addictions registered nurse and the graduate-level prepared addictions registered nurse, the addictions advanced practice registered nurse:

- Initiates and interprets diagnostic tests and procedures relevant to the healthcare consumer's current status.
- Uses advanced assessment, knowledge, and skills to maintain, enhance, or improve health conditions.

STANDARD 2. DIAGNOSIS

The addictions registered nurse analyzes the assessment data to determine actual or potential diagnoses, problems, and issues.

Competencies

The addictions registered nurse:

- Identifies actual or potential risks to the healthcare consumer's health and safety or barriers to health, which may include but are not limited to interpersonal, systematic, cultural, or environmental circumstances.
- Identifies the behavioral, psychological, physical health, and social effects of psychoactive substances on the person using and significant others.
- Recognizes the potential for substance use disorders to mimic a variety of medical and mental health conditions and the potential for medical and mental health conditions to coexist with substance use and addiction.
- Verifies the diagnoses, problems, and issues with the individual, family, group, community, population, and interprofessional colleagues.
- Prioritizes diagnoses, problems, and issues based on mutually established goals to meet the needs of the healthcare consumer across the health-illness continuum.
- Uses assessment data, standardized classification systems, technology, and clinical decision support tools to articulate actual or potential diagnoses, problems, and issues.
- Documents diagnoses, problems, and issues in a manner that facilitates the determination of the expected outcomes and plan.

ADDITIONAL COMPETENCIES FOR THE GRADUATE-LEVEL PREPARED REGISTERED NURSE IN THE ADDICTIONS SPECIALTY

In addition to the competencies of the addictions registered nurse, the graduate-level prepared addictions registered nurse:

- Uses information and communication technologies to analyze practice patterns of nurses and other members of the interprofessional healthcare team.

- Employs aggregate-level data to articulate diagnoses, problems, issues of healthcare consumers, and organizational systems.

ADDITIONAL COMPETENCIES FOR THE ADVANCED PRACTICE REGISTERED NURSE IN THE ADDICTIONS SPECIALTY

In addition to the competencies of the addictions registered nurse and the graduate-level prepared addictions registered nurse, the addictions advanced practice registered nurse:

- Formulates a differential diagnosis based on the assessment, history, physical examination, and diagnostic test results.

STANDARD 3. OUTCOMES IDENTIFICATION

The registered nurse specializing in addictions identifies expected outcomes for a plan individualized to the healthcare consumer or the situation.

Competencies

The addictions registered nurse:

- Engages the healthcare consumer, interprofessional team, and others in partnership to identify expected outcomes.
- Understands the importance of research and outcome data and their application in clinical practice.
- Formulates evidence-based and culturally sensitive outcomes derived from the assessment and identified diagnoses.
- Develops expected outcomes that facilitate coordination of care.
- Uses clinical expertise and current evidence-based practices to identify risks, benefits, costs, and/or expected trajectory of the condition.
- Collaborates with the healthcare consumer to define expected outcomes integrating the healthcare consumer's culture, values, and ethical considerations.
- Generates a timeframe for the attainment of expected outcomes.
- Modifies expected outcomes based on evaluation of the status of the healthcare consumer and situation.

- Documents expected outcomes as measurable goals.
- Evaluates the actual outcomes in relation to expected outcomes, safety, and quality standards.

ADDITIONAL COMPETENCIES FOR THE GRADUATE-LEVEL PREPARED REGISTERED NURSE, INCLUDING THE ADVANCED PRACTICE REGISTERED NURSE IN THE ADDICTIONS SPECIALTY

In addition to the competencies of the addictions registered nurse, the graduate-level prepared addictions registered nurse or advanced practice registered addictions nurse:

- Defines expected outcomes that incorporate costs and clinical effectiveness and are aligned with the outcomes identified by members of the interprofessional team.
- Differentiates outcomes that require process interventions from those that require system-level actions.
- Integrates scientific evidence and implements practice changes to achieve expected outcomes.
- Advocates for outcomes that reflect the healthcare consumer's culture, values, and ethical considerations.

STANDARD 4. PLANNING

The addictions registered nurse develops a plan that prescribes strategies to attain expected, measurable outcomes.

Competencies

The addictions registered nurse:

- Develops an individualized, holistic, evidence-based plan in partnership with the healthcare consumer and interprofessional team.
- Values an interdisciplinary approach to addiction treatment.
- Establishes priorities with the healthcare consumer and interprofessional team.

- Advocates for responsible and appropriate use of intervention to minimize unwarranted or unwanted treatment and/or healthcare consumer suffering.
- Prioritizes elements of the plan based on the assessment of the healthcare consumer's level of risk and safety needs.
- Includes evidence-based strategies in the plan to address each of the identified diagnoses, problems, or issues. These strategies may include, but are not limited to, strategies for the following:
    - Promotion and restoration of health;
    - Prevention of illness, injury, and disease;
    - Facilitation of healing;
    - Alleviation of suffering; and
    - Supportive care.
- Tailors helping strategies and treatment modalities to the severity of the substance use, the consumer's readiness to change, the availability of treatment resources, and the consumer's anticipated recovery outcomes.
- Includes strategies for health, wholeness, and recovery across the lifespan.
- Incorporates an implementation pathway that describes steps and milestones.
- Identifies the availability of treatment and recovery services, insurance benefits, the costs and economic implications of implementing the treatment plan, and the importance of helping consumers to access services and benefits.
- Develops a plan that reflects compliance with current statutes, rules and regulations, and standards.
- Modifies the plan according to the ongoing assessment of the healthcare consumer's response and other outcome indicators.
- Documents the plan in a manner that uses standardized recovery-oriented, nonstigmatizing language and recognized terminology.

In addition to the competencies of the addictions registered nurse, the graduate-level prepared addictions registered nurse:

- Designs strategies and tactics to meet the complex and multidimensional needs of healthcare consumers.
- Leads the design and development of interprofessional processes to address the identified diagnoses, problems, or issues.
- Integrates assessment and diagnostic with therapeutic interventions to reflect current evidence-based knowledge and practice.
- Designs innovative nursing practices.
- Actively participates in the development and continuous improvement of systems that support the planning process.

STANDARD 5. IMPLEMENTATION

The addictions registered nurse implements the identified plan.

Competencies

The addictions registered nurse:

- Partners with the healthcare consumer to implement the plan in a safe, effective, efficient, timely, patient-centered, and equitable manner (Institute of Medicine [IOM], 2001, 2006, 2011).
- Based on the initial action plan, takes specific steps to initiate an admission or referral and ensure follow-through.
- Integrates interprofessional team partners in implementation of the plan through collaboration and communication across the continuum of care.
- Demonstrates caring behaviors to develop therapeutic relationships.
- Provides culturally congruent, holistic care.
- Advocates for the needs of diverse populations across the lifespan.

- Uses evidence-based interventions and strategies to achieve mutually identified goals and outcomes specific to the problem or needs.
- Informs the healthcare consumer of confidentiality rights, program procedures that safeguard them, and the exceptions imposed by regulations.
- Integrates critical thinking and technology solutions to implement the nursing process to collect, measure, record, retrieve, trend, and analyze data and information to enhance nursing practice and healthcare consumer outcomes.
- Appropriately delegates according to the health, safety, and welfare needs of the healthcare consumer.
- Maintains accountability for care, with consideration of state nurse practice act and other regulations.
- Reassesses the treatment plan at regular intervals or when indicated by changing circumstances.
- Documents implementation and any modifications, including changes or omissions, of the identified plan.

ADDITIONAL COMPETENCIES FOR THE GRADUATE-LEVEL PREPARED REGISTERED NURSE IN THE ADDICTIONS SPECIALTY

In addition to the competencies of the addictions registered nurse, the graduate-level prepared addictions registered nurse:

- Uses systems, organizations, and community resources to lead effective change.
- Applies quality principles while articulating methods, tools, performance measures, and standards as they relate to implementation of the plan.
- Translates evidence into practice.
- Leads interprofessional teams to communicate, collaborate, and consult effectively.
- Demonstrates leadership skills that emphasize ethical and critical decision-making, effective working relationships, and a systems perspective.

- Serves as a consultant to provide additional insight and potential solutions.
- Uses theory-driven approaches to effect organizational or system change.

Additional Competencies for the Advanced Practice Registered Nurse in the Addictions Specialty

In addition to the competencies of the addictions registered nurse and the graduate-level prepared addictions registered nurse, the addictions advanced practice registered nurse:

- Uses prescriptive authority, procedures, referrals, treatments, and therapies in accordance with state and federal laws and regulations.
- Prescribes traditional and integrative evidence-based treatments, therapies, and procedures that are compatible with professional standards of care as well as the healthcare consumer's preferences.
- Prescribes evidence-based pharmacologic, behavioral, and other treatments according to all scope of practice and regulatory requirements, as well as clinical indicators and results of diagnostic and laboratory tests.
- Provides clinical consultation related to complex clinical cases for improved care and patient outcomes.

STANDARD 5A. COORDINATION OF CARE

The addictions registered nurse coordinates care delivery, programs, services, and other activities as needed to implement the identified plan.

Competencies

The addictions registered nurse:

- Collaborates with the healthcare consumer to identify treatment options.
- Coordinates components of the plan to reach mutually agreed-upon outcomes.

- Engages healthcare consumers in self-care to achieve preferred goals for quality of life.
- Arranges appropriate referrals to other professionals, agencies, community programs, or resources to meet the client's needs.
- Communicates in clear and specific language to help the consumer follow through with the referral and safely transition within the care continuum.
- Advocates for the delivery of dignified, humane, and holistic care by the interprofessional team.
- Documents the coordination and receipt of care.
- Continuously assesses and evaluates referral resources to determine their appropriateness.

ADDITIONAL COMPETENCIES FOR THE GRADUATE-LEVEL PREPARED REGISTERED NURSE IN THE ADDICTIONS SPECIALTY

In addition to the competencies of the addictions registered nurse, the graduate-level prepared addictions registered nurse:

- Provides leadership in the coordination of interprofessional health care for integrated delivery of healthcare consumer services to achieve safe, effective, efficient, timely, patient-centered, and equitable care (IOM, 2011).

ADDITIONAL COMPETENCIES FOR THE ADVANCED PRACTICE REGISTERED NURSE IN THE ADDICTIONS SPECIALTY

In addition to the competencies of the addictions registered nurse and the graduate-level prepared addictions registered nurse, the addictions advanced practice registered nurse:

- Manages identified consumer panels or populations.
- Serves as the healthcare consumer's primary care provider and coordinator of healthcare services in accordance with state and federal laws and regulations.
- Synthesizes information to prescribe and provide necessary system and community support measures.

STANDARD 5B. HEALTH TEACHING AND HEALTH PROMOTION

The addictions registered nurse employs strategies to promote health and a safe environment.

Competencies

The addictions registered nurse:

- Provides opportunities for the healthcare consumer to identify needed health promotion, disease prevention, recovery support, and self-management topics.
- Incorporates the consumer's values, beliefs, health practices, developmental level, learning needs, readiness and ability to learn, language preference, spirituality, culture, and socioeconomic status into health promotion and health teaching methods.
- Solicits feedback and the consumer's perspectives to determine the effectiveness of strategies employed.
- Uses technologies to communicate health promotion and disease prevention information to the healthcare consumer.
- Provides anticipatory guidance to healthcare consumers to promote health and prevent or reduce the risk of negative health outcomes.
- Provides information about intended effects and potential adverse effects of planned interventions.
- Provides healthcare consumers with information about potential beneficial outcomes and side effects of medications for the treatment of psychiatric and mental health conditions and substance use disorders.
- Engages consumer alliance and advocacy groups in health teaching and health promotion activities for healthcare consumers.
- Provides information about the definition of a standard drink, safe drinking limits, and risky alcohol use.
- Reinforces that no amount of alcohol or illicit drug is safe for women who are pregnant or intending to become pregnant.

- Advises on the risks associated with substance use and risk behaviors for high-risk individuals (e.g., adolescents, pregnant women, those with comorbid medical and mental disorders).
- Provides endorsed educational material related to substance use and other addictive disorders (e.g., from IntNSA, Department of Veterans Affairs, National Institute on Alcohol Abuse and Alcoholism, NIDA, Substance Abuse and Mental Health Administration Services).

ADDITIONAL COMPETENCIES FOR THE GRADUATE-LEVEL PREPARED REGISTERED NURSE, INCLUDING THE ADVANCED PRACTICE REGISTERED NURSE IN THE ADDICTIONS SPECIALTY

In addition to the competencies of the addictions registered nurse, the graduate-level prepared addictions registered nurse or addictions advanced practice registered nurse:

- Synthesizes empirical evidence on risk behaviors, gender roles, learning theories, behavioral change theories, motivational theories, translational theories for evidence-based practice, epidemiology, and other related theories and frameworks when designing health education information and programs.
- Evaluates health information resources for applicability, accuracy, readability, and comprehensibility to help consumers access quality health information.

STANDARD 6. EVALUATION

The addictions registered nurse evaluates progress toward attainment of goals and outcomes.

Competencies

The addictions registered nurse:

- Uses ongoing assessment data and synthesizes information to revise the diagnoses, outcomes, plan, and implementation strategies.

- Collaborates with the healthcare consumer and others involved when evaluating and modifying the plan of care.
- Conducts a holistic, systematic, and criterion-based evaluation of attainment of goals and outcomes in relation to the structure, processes, and timeline prescribed in the plan.
- Determines, in partnership with the consumer, the patient-centeredness, effectiveness, efficiency, safety, timeliness, equitability, quality, and safety of the plan (IOM, 2001; Kelly et al., 2018).
- Shares evaluation data and conclusions with the healthcare consumer and other stakeholders in accordance with federal and state regulations.
- Documents the results of the evaluation.

ADDITIONAL COMPETENCIES FOR THE GRADUATE-LEVEL PREPARED REGISTERED NURSE, INCLUDING THE ADVANCED PRACTICE REGISTERED NURSE IN THE ADDICTIONS SPECIALTY

In addition to the competencies of the addictions registered nurse, the graduate-level prepared addictions registered nurse or addictions advanced practice registered nurse:

- Uses results of the consumer and provider evaluations to make or recommend process, policy, procedure, or protocol revisions when warranted.

Standards of Professional Performance for Addictions Nursing

STANDARD 7. ETHICS

The addictions registered nurse practices ethically.

Competencies

The addictions registered nurse:

- Integrates the *Code of Ethics for Nurses With Interpretive Statements* (American Nurses Association [ANA], 2015a) to guide nursing practice and articulate the moral foundation of nursing.
- Practices with compassion and respect for the inherent dignity, worth, and unique attributes of all people.
- Advocates for healthcare consumers' rights to informed decision-making and self-determination.
- Seeks guidance in situations where the rights of the individual conflict with public health guidelines.
- Endorses the understanding that the primary commitment is to the healthcare consumer regardless of setting or situation.
- Maintains therapeutic relationships and professional boundaries.
- Advocates for the rights, health, and safety of the healthcare consumer and others.

- Safeguards the privacy and confidentiality of healthcare consumers and others and of their data and information within ethical, legal, and regulatory parameters.
- Upholds healthcare consumer confidentiality within legal and regulatory parameters, including the Health Insurance Portability and Accountability Act (HIPAA, 1996) and strict adherence to the Code of Federal Regulations, Confidentiality of Substance Use Disorder Patient Records (42 C.F.R. Part 2; 2017).
- Demonstrates professional accountability and responsibility for nursing practice.
- Maintains competence through continued personal and professional development.
- Demonstrates commitment to self-reflection and self-care.
- Contributes to the establishment and maintenance of an ethical environment that is conducive to safe, quality health care.
- Establishes a sustained culture of respect, free of incivility, bullying, and workplace violence.
- Maintains an ethical environment and culture of civility and kindness by treating colleagues, coworkers, employees, students, and others with dignity and respect.
- Advances the profession through scholarly inquiry, professional standards development, and the generation of policy.
- Collaborates with other health professionals and the public to protect human rights, promote health diplomacy, enhance cultural sensitivity and congruence, and reduce health disparities.
- Articulates nursing values to maintain personal integrity and the integrity of the profession.
- Integrates principles of social justice into nursing and policy.

STANDARD 8. CULTURALLY CONGRUENT PRACTICE

The addictions registered nurse practices in a manner that is congruent with cultural diversity and inclusion principles.

Competencies

The addictions registered nurse:

- Demonstrates respect, equity, empathy, and cultural humility in actions and interactions with all healthcare consumers.
- Participates in lifelong learning to understand cultural preferences, worldviews, choices, and decision-making processes of diverse consumers.
- Creates an inventory of one's own values, beliefs, and cultural heritage.
- Applies knowledge of variations in health beliefs, practices, and communication patterns in all nursing practice activities.
- Identifies the stage of the healthcare consumer's acculturation and accompanying patterns of needs and engagement.
- Considers the effects and impact of discrimination and oppression on practice within and among vulnerable cultural groups.
- Uses skills and tools that are appropriately vetted for the culture, literacy, and language of the population served.
- Communicates with appropriate language and behaviors including the use of medical interpreters and translators in accordance with consumer preferences.
- Identifies the cultural-specific meaning of interactions, terms, and content.
- Respects consumer decisions based on age, tradition, belief, family influence, and stage of acculturation.
- Advocates for policies that promote health and prevent harm among culturally diverse, underserved, or underrepresented consumers.
- Promotes equal access to services, tests, interventions, health promotion programs, enrollment in research, education, and other opportunities.
- Educates nurse colleagues and other professionals about cultural similarities and differences of healthcare consumers, families, groups, communities, and populations.

ADDITIONAL COMPETENCIES FOR THE GRADUATE-LEVEL PREPARED REGISTERED NURSE IN THE ADDICTIONS SPECIALTY

In addition to the competencies of the addictions registered nurse, the graduate-level prepared addictions registered nurse:

- Evaluates tools, instruments, and services provided to culturally diverse populations.
- Advances organizational policies, programs, services, and practices that reflect respect, equity, diversity, and inclusion.
- Engages consumers, key stakeholders, and others in designing and establishing internal and external cross-cultural partnerships.
- Conducts research to improve health care and healthcare outcomes for culturally diverse consumers.
- Develops recruitment and retention strategies to achieve a multicultural workforce.

ADDITIONAL COMPETENCIES FOR THE ADVANCED PRACTICE REGISTERED NURSE IN THE ADDICTIONS SPECIALTY

In addition to the competencies of the addictions registered nurse and the graduate-level prepared addictions registered nurse, the advanced practice addictions registered nurse:

- Promotes shared problem-solving approaches and decision-making solutions in planning, prescribing, and evaluation processes when the healthcare consumer's preferences, values, and norms create incompatibility with safe nursing practice.
- Leads interprofessional teams to ensure that clinical care provided incorporates the cultural and language needs of consumers.

STANDARD 9. COMMUNICATION

The addictions registered nurse communicates effectively in all areas of practice.

Competencies

The addictions registered nurse:

- Assesses one's own communication skills and effectiveness.
- Demonstrates cultural empathy when communicating.
- Assesses communication ability, health literacy, resources, and preferences of healthcare consumers to inform the interprofessional team and others.
- Adheres to the *National Standards for Culturally and Linguistically Appropriate Services* (CLAS).
- Uses preferred language or language translation resources to ensure effective written and oral communications.
- Incorporates appropriate alternative strategies to communicate effectively with healthcare consumers who have visual, speech, language, or communication difficulty.
- Uses communication styles and methods that demonstrate caring, respect, deep listening, authenticity, and trust.
- Conveys accurate information.
- Maintains communication with other interprofessional teams and others to facilitate safe transitions and continuity in care delivery.
- Contributes the nursing perspective in interactions with others and discussions with the interprofessional team.
- Exposes care processes and decisions when they do not appear to be in the best interest of the healthcare consumer.
- Discloses concerns related to potential or actual hazards and errors in care or the practice environment to the appropriate level.
- Demonstrates continuous improvement of communication skills.

In addition to the competencies of the addictions registered nurse, the graduate-level prepared addictions registered nurse or advanced practice registered nurse:

- Assumes a leadership role in shaping or fashioning environments that promote healthy communication.

STANDARD 10. COLLABORATION

The addictions registered nurse collaborates with the healthcare consumer and other key stakeholders in the conduct of nursing practice.

Competencies

The addictions registered nurse:

- Clearly articulates the nurse's role, responsibilities, and identified areas of expertise and contribution within the healthcare team.
- Utilizes core competencies for interprofessional collaborative practice and team-based care.
- Incorporates effective group dynamics, effective communication skills, consensus building, conflict management, and other strategies to enhance team performance.
- Optimizes the unique and complementary abilities of all members of the team to optimize attainment of desired outcomes.
- Uses appropriate tools and techniques, including information systems and technologies, to facilitate discussion and team functions, in a manner that protects dignity, respect, privacy, and confidentiality.
- Exhibits dignity, civility, and respect when interacting with others and giving and receiving feedback.

- Partners with all stakeholders to create, implement, modify, and evaluate delivery of comprehensive quality care.

ADDITIONAL COMPETENCIES FOR THE GRADUATE-LEVEL PREPARED REGISTERED NURSE, INCLUDING THE ADVANCED PRACTICE REGISTERED NURSE IN THE ADDICTIONS SPECIALTY

In addition to the competencies of the addictions registered nurse, the graduate-level prepared addictions nurse or the advanced practice registered nurse:

- Participates in interprofessional activities, including but not limited to education, consultation, management, technological development, and research to enhance outcomes.
- Provides leadership for establishing, improving, and sustaining collaborative relationships to achieve safe, quality care for healthcare consumers.
- Advances interprofessional plan-of-care documentation and communications, rationales for plan-of-care changes, and collaborative discussions to improve healthcare consumer outcomes.

STANDARD 11. LEADERSHIP

The addictions registered nurse leads within the professional practice setting and the profession.

Competencies

The addictions registered nurse:

- Contributes to the establishment of an environment that supports and maintains civility, respect, trust, and dignity (ANA, n.d.-c).

- Maintains a safe and healthy work environment by prohibiting workplace incivility and bullying (ANA, n.d.-c).
- Incorporates appropriate safety measures to prevent workplace violence.
- Encourages innovation in practice and role performance to obtain personal and professional plans, goals, and vision.
- Communicates to manage change and address conflict.
- Mentors colleagues for the advancement of nursing practice and the profession to enhance safe, quality health care.
- Retains accountability for delegated nursing care.
- Promote acculturation of nurses who are new to their roles by role modeling, orienting, mentoring, encouraging, providing emotional and material supports, and sharing pertinent information relative to optimal care delivery.
- Contributes to the evolution of the profession through participation in professional organizations.
- Influences policy to promote health.

ADDITIONAL COMPETENCIES FOR THE GRADUATE-LEVEL PREPARED REGISTERED NURSE, INCLUDING THE ADVANCED PRACTICE REGISTERED NURSE IN THE ADDICTIONS SPECIALTY

In addition to the competencies of the registered nurse, the graduate-level prepared addictions nurse or the advanced practice registered nurse:

- Influences decision-making bodies to improve the professional practice environment and healthcare consumer outcomes.
- Enhances the effectiveness of the interprofessional team.
- Promotes advanced practice nursing and role development by interpreting its role for healthcare consumers and policymakers.
- Models expert practice.
- Mentors nursing and interprofessional colleagues in the acquisition of clinical knowledge, skills, abilities, and judgment.

STANDARD 12. EDUCATION

The addictions registered nurse seeks knowledge and competence that reflects current nursing practice and promotes futuristic thinking.

Competencies

The addictions registered nurse:

- Identifies learning needs of self and others based on nursing knowledge and the various roles nurses may assume.
- Seeks experiences that reflect current practice to maintain and advance knowledge, skills, abilities, attitudes, and judgment in clinical practice or role performance.
- Acquires knowledge and skills relative to the role, population, specialty, setting, and global or local health situation.
- Participates in ongoing educational activities related to nursing and interprofessional knowledge bases and professional topics.
- Demonstrates a commitment to lifelong learning through self-reflection and inquiry for learning and personal growth.
- Participates in formal consultations or informal discussion to address issues in nursing practice as an application of education and knowledge.
- Incorporates modifications and/or accommodations needed in the delivery of consumer and family education.
- Disseminates educational findings, experiences, and ideas with peers.
- Facilitates a work environment supportive of ongoing education of healthcare professionals.
- Maintains a professional portfolio that provides evidence of individual competence and lifelong learning.
- Promotes addictions-related knowledge (e.g., screening, brief intervention, and referral to treatment [SBIRT]; medications for substance use disorder treatment; motivational interviewing; other treatment modalities) by sharing with interprofessional colleagues and nurses in other specialties.

STANDARD 13. EVIDENCE-BASED PRACTICE AND RESEARCH

The addictions registered nurse integrates evidence and research findings into practice.

Competencies

The addictions registered nurse:

- Utilizes evidence-based practice guidelines and standardized technical applications in situations where outcomes are predictable and reliable.
- Utilizes sound reasoning, clinical judgment, and nursing expertise when a particular individual exhibits an uncharacteristic response.
- Utilizes theory to explain certain phenomena and relationships between associated concepts or to predict causal relationships that can lead to specific events or outcomes, in order to improve the quality and safety of care.
- Articulates the values of research and its application relative to the healthcare settings and practice.
- Identifies practice questions in the healthcare setting that can be answered by nursing and other health research.
- Appraises nursing and other health research methods and outcomes in order to incorporate evidence-based interventions when initiating nursing practice changes.
- Evaluates achievement of outcomes against those found in nursing and other research.
- Uses clinical expertise based on current evidence-based research findings, as well as the consumer's preferences, values, and health data to guide practice.
- Participates in the formulation of evidence-based practice through research.
- Promotes ethical principles of research in practice and the healthcare setting.
- Disseminates peer-reviewed research findings with colleagues to integrate knowledge into nursing practice.

In addition to the competencies of the addictions registered nurse, the graduate-level prepared addictions nurse or the advanced practice registered nurse:

- Integrates research-based practice in all settings.
- Uses current research findings and other evidence to expand knowledge, skills, abilities, and judgment; to enhance role performance; and to increase knowledge of professional issues.
- Utilizes quality improvement (QI) process models to assess, plan, and implement evidence-based practice changes.
- Performs systematic appraisal and rigorous critique of research to generate meaningful evidence for nursing practice.
- Develops research and implementation science skills in order to develop and implement evidence-based practice changes and disseminate research findings and implementation processes, barriers, and facilitators.
- Promotes a climate of collaborative research and clinical inquiry.
- Advocates for the ethical conduct of research and translational scholarship with particular attention to the protection of the healthcare consumer as a research participant.

STANDARD 14. QUALITY OF PRACTICE

The addictions registered nurse contributes to quality nursing practice.

Competencies

The addictions registered nurse:

- Ensures that addictions nursing practice is safe, effective, efficient, equitable, timely, and patient-centered (Institute of Medicine [IOM], 2001, 2006).

- Identifies barriers, facilitators, and opportunities and recommends strategies to improve the quality of health care.
- Establishes rapport, including management of a crisis situation and determination of need for additional professional assistance.
- Collects data to monitor the quality of nursing practice.
- Contributes in efforts to improve healthcare efficiency.
- Uses creativity and innovation to enhance nursing care.
- Participates in quality improvement initiatives.
- Provides critical review and/or evaluation of policies, procedures, and guidelines to improve the quality of health care.
- Engages in formal and informal peer review processes.
- Collaborates with the interprofessional team to implement quality improvement plans and interventions.
- Documents addictions nursing practice in a manner that supports quality and performance improvement initiatives.
- Achieves professional certification such as the Certified Addictions Registered Nurse (CARN) and the Certified Addictions Registered Nurse-Advanced Practice (CARN-AP).

ADDITIONAL COMPETENCIES FOR THE GRADUATE-LEVEL PREPARED REGISTERED NURSE

In addition to the competencies for the addictions registered nurse, the graduate-level prepared addictions nurse:

- Analyzes trends in healthcare quality data, including examination of cultural influences and factors.
- Provides leadership in the design and implementation of quality improvement initiatives.
- Implements innovative practice changes to improve outcomes.
- Contributes to addictions nursing and interprofessional knowledge through scientific inquiry.
- Influences the organizational system and promotes a practice environment that supports evidence-based health care and improved outcomes.

- Engages in development, implementation, evaluation, and/or revision of policies, procedures, and guidelines to improve healthcare quality.
- Uses data and information in systems-level decision-making.
- Encourages professional and/or specialty certification.

ADDITIONAL COMPETENCIES FOR THE ADVANCED PRACTICE REGISTERED NURSE IN THE ADDICTIONS SPECIALTY

In addition to the competencies for the addictions registered nurse and the graduate-level prepared addictions nurse, the advanced practice registered nurse:

- Engages in comparison evaluation of the effectiveness and efficacy of diagnostic tests, clinical procedures and therapies, and treatment plans, in partnership with healthcare consumers to optimize health, healthcare quality, and recovery.
- Uses available benchmarks as a means to evaluate practice at the individual, departmental, or organizational level.

STANDARD 15. PROFESSIONAL PRACTICE EVALUATION

The addictions registered nurse evaluates one's own and others' nursing practice.

Competencies

The addictions registered nurse:

- Adheres to the guidance about professional practice as specified in the *Nursing: Scope and Standards of Practice* and the *Code of Ethics for Nurses with Interpretive Statements*.
- Ensures that addictions nursing practice is consistent with regulatory requirements pertaining to licensure, relevant statutes, rules, and regulations.

- Uses organizational policies and procedures to guide professional practice.
- Influences organizational policies and procedures to promote interprofessional evidence-based practice.
- Engages in lifelong learning, self-reflection, and self-evaluation to identify areas of strength as well as areas in which professional growth would be beneficial.
- Seeks formal and informal feedback regarding one's own practice from healthcare consumers, peers, colleagues, supervisors, and others.
- Provides peers and others with formal and informal constructive feedback regarding their practice or role performance.
- Takes action to achieve goals identified during the evaluation process.

STANDARD 16. RESOURCE UTILIZATION

The addictions registered nurse utilizes appropriate resources to plan, provide, and sustain evidence-based nursing services that are safe, effective, and fiscally responsible.

Competencies

The addictions registered nurse:

- Assesses individual healthcare consumer care needs, coordinates care, and provides linkages to available organizational and community-based resources to achieve desired outcomes.
- Assists the healthcare consumer in identifying and securing appropriate services to address needs across the healthcare continuum.
- Assists the healthcare consumer in factoring costs, risks, and benefits in decisions about care.
- Identifies impact of resource allocation on the potential for harm, complexity of the task, and desired outcomes.
- Advocates for resources that support and enhance nursing practice.

- Delegates in accordance with applicable legal and policy parameters.
- Integrates telehealth and mobile health technologies into practice to remove barriers and improve access to care.
- Addresses discriminatory healthcare practices and their impact on resource allocation and access to care.

ADDITIONAL COMPETENCIES FOR THE GRADUATE-LEVEL PREPARED REGISTERED NURSE IN THE ADDICTIONS SPECIALTY

In addition to the competencies of the addictions registered nurse, the graduate-level prepared addictions nurse:

- Assumes complex and advanced leadership roles to initiate and guide change.
- Designs innovative solutions such as systems integration initiatives and collaborative care models to promote effective resource utilization, continuity of care, and healthcare quality.
- Expands addictions treatment capacity and improves access to prevention and treatment services through grant writing, program development, and advocacy.
- Creates evaluation strategies that address cost effectiveness, cost benefit, and efficiency factors associated with addictions nursing practice.

ADDITIONAL COMPETENCIES FOR THE ADVANCED PRACTICE REGISTERED NURSE IN THE ADDICTIONS SPECIALTY

In addition to the competencies of the addictions registered nurse and the graduate-level prepared addictions nurse, the addictions advanced practice registered nurse:

- Improves access to high-quality care that addresses unmet healthcare needs of consumers in underserved areas, both urban and rural.

STANDARD 17. ENVIRONMENTAL HEALTH

The addictions registered nurse practices in an environmentally safe and healthy manner.

Competencies

The addictions registered nurse:

- Promotes a safe and healthy workplace and professional practice environment.
- Utilizes environmental health concepts and technologies.
- Assesses the environment to identify risk factors and reduce environmental health risks to self, colleagues, and healthcare consumers (ANA, n.d.-c).
- Applies setting-specific policies and procedures for handling crisis or dangerous situations, including safety measures for clients and staff.
- Communicates information about environmental health risks and exposure reduction strategies.
- Advocates for the safe, judicious, and appropriate disposal of products in health care.
- Uses products or treatments consistent with evidence-based practice to reduce environmental threats.
- Participates in developing strategies to promote healthy communities and practice environments.

ADDITIONAL COMPETENCIES FOR THE GRADUATE-LEVEL PREPARED REGISTERED NURSE, INCLUDING THE ADVANCED PRACTICE REGISTERED NURSE IN THE ADDICTIONS SPECIALTY

In addition to the competencies of the addictions registered nurse, the graduate-level prepared addictions nurse and advanced practice registered nurse:

- Analyzes the impact of social, political, and economic influences on the global environment and human health experience.

- Creates partnerships that promote sustainable global environmental health policies and conditions that focus on prevention of hazards to people and the natural environment (ANA, 2007).

References

Abraham, A. J., Riechmann, T., Andrews, C. M., & Jayawardhana, J. (2017). Health insurance enrollment and availability of medications for substance use disorders. *Psychiatric Services*, 68(1), 41–47.

Ahmedani, B. (2011). Mental health stigma: Society, individual and the profession. *Journal of Social Work Values and Ethics*, 8(2) 4-1-4-16. https://www.ncbi.nlm.nih.gov/pmc/articles/PMC3248273/pdf/nihms342711.pdf

American Academy of Addiction Psychiatry. (2015, May). *Relationship between treatment and self-help*. https://www.aaap.org/wp-content/uploads/2015/06/Relat-bw-Treatment-SelfHelp-1997.pdf

American Association of Colleges of Nursing. (2006, October). *The essentials of doctoral education for advanced nursing practice*. https://www.aacnnursing.org/Portals/42/Publications/DNPEssentials.pdf

American Association of Colleges of Nursing. (2010). *Research-focused doctoral program in nursing: Pathways to excellence*. https://www.aacnnursing.org/Portals/42/Publications/PhDPosition.pdf

American Association of Colleges of Nursing. (2011, March 21). *The essentials of master's education in nursing*. https://www.aacnnursing.org/Portals/42/Publications/MastersEssentials11.pdf

American Association of Colleges of Nursing. (2019). *Academic progression in nursing: Moving together toward a highly educated nursing workforce*. https://www.aacnnursing.org/News-Information/Position-Statements-White-Papers/Academic-Progression-in-Nursing

American Association of Colleges of Nursing. (2021, April 6). *The essentials: Core competencies for professional nursing education*. https://www.aacnnursing.org/Portals/42/AcademicNursing/pdf/Essentials-2021.pdf

American Geriatrics Society Beers Criteria® Update Expert Panel. (2019). American Geriatrics Society 2019 updated AGS Beers Criteria® for potentially inappropriate medication use in older adults. *Journal of the American Geriatrics Society*, 67(4), 674–694. https://doi.org/10.1111/jgs.15767

American Nurses Association. (n.d.-a). *About ANA*. https://epicmsdev.nursingworld.org/ana/about-ana/

American Nurses Association. (n.d.-b). *Advanced practice registered nurse (APRN)*. https://www.nursingworld.org/practice-policy/workforce/what-is-nursing/aprn/

American Nurses Association. (n.d.-c) *Healthy work environment*. https://www.nursingworld.org/practice-policy/work-environment/

American Nurses Association. (2007). *ANA principles of environmental health for nursing practice with implementation strategies*. Silver Spring, MD.

American Nurses Association. (2014). *Professional role competence: ANA position statement.* https://www.nursingworld.org/practice-policy/nursing-excellence/official-position-statements/id/professional-role-competence/

American Nurses Association. (2015a). *Code of ethics for nurses with interpretive statements* (2nd ed.). Silver Spring, MD.

American Nurses Association. (2015b). *Nursing: Scope and standards of practice* (3rd ed.). Silver Spring, MD.

American Nurses Association. (2017). *American Nurses Association strongly opposes the new health care reform bill.* https://www.nursingworld.org/news/news-releases/2020/ana-calls-administrations--court-filing-to-overturn-the-affordable-care-act-unconscionable/

American Nurses Association Ethics Advisory Board. (2018, October 29). ANA position statement: The ethical responsibility to manage pain and the suffering it causes. *Online Journal of Issues in Nursing, 24*(1). https://doi.org/10.3912/OJIN.Vol24No01PoSCol01

American Nurses Association, International Nurses Society on Addictions, & Drug and Alcohol Nurses Association. (1987). *Care of clients with addictions: Dimensions of nursing practice.*

American Psychiatric Association. (2013). *Diagnostic and statistical manual of mental disorders* (5th ed.). https://doi.org/10.1176/appi.books.9780890425596

American Psychological Association. (2012). Building your resilience. https://www.apa.org/topics/resilience

American Society of Addiction Medicine. (2011, August 15). *Public policy statement: Definition of addiction.* https://www.asam.org/docs/default-source/public-policy-statements/1definition_of_addiction_long_4-11.pdf?sfvrsn=a8f64512_4

American Society of Addiction Medicine. (2015, May 13). *ASAM continuum knowledge base: What are the ASAM levels of care?* https://www.asamcontinuum.org/knowledgebase/what-are-the-asam-levels-of-care/

American Society of Addiction Medicine. (2017). *Appropriate use of drug testing in clinical addiction medicine.* https://www.asam.org/Quality-Science/quality/drug-testing

American Society of Addiction Medicine. (2019, September 15). *Definition of addiction.* https://www.asam.org/docs/default-source/quality-science/asam's-2019-definition-of-addiction-(1).pdf?sfvrsn=b8b64fc2_2

Amnesty International. (n.d.). *LGBTQI glossary.* https://www.amnestyusa.org/pdfs/AIUSA_Pride2015Glossary.pdf

APRN Consensus Work Group & National Council of State Boards of Nursing APRN Advisory Committee. (2008, July 7). *Consensus model for APRN regulation: Licensure, accreditation, certification and education.* https://www.nursingworld.org/~4aa7d9/globalassets/certification/aprn_consensus_model_report_7-7-08.pdf

Austin, A. E., Proescholdbell, S. K., Creppage, K. E., & Asbun, A. (2017). Characteristics of self-inflicted drug overdose deaths in North Carolina. *Drug and Alcohol Dependence, 181,* 44–49. https://doi.org/10.1016/j.drugalcdep.2017.09.014

Babor, T. F., & Higgins-Biddle, J. C. (2001). *Brief interventions for harmful and hazardous alcohol use: A manual for use in primary care.* http://apps.who.int/iris/bitstream/10665/67210/1/WHO_MSD_MSB_01.6b.pdf

Babor, T. F., Higgins-Biddle, J. C., Saunders, J. B., & Monteiro, M. G. (2001). *The Alcohol Use Disorders Identification Test (AUDIT): Guidelines for use in primary care.* http://whqlibdoc.who.int/hq/2001/WHO_MSD_MSB_01.6a.pdf

Babor, T. F., Ritson, E. B., & Hodgson, R. J. (1986). Alcohol-related problems in the primary health care setting: A review of early intervention strategies. *British Journal of Addiction, 81*(1), 23–46. https://doi.org/10.1111/j.1360-0443.1986.tb00291.x

Bailey, P. (2017). *ACA repeal would jeopardize treatment for millions with substance use disorders, including opioid addiction.* Center on Budget and Policy Priorities. http://www.cbpp.org/sites/default/files/atoms/files/2-9-17health.pdf

Bennett, G., Vourakis, C., & Woolf, D. S. (Eds.). (1983) *Substance abuse: Pharmacologic, developmental, and clinical perspectives.* John Wiley & Sons.

Biederman, J., Faraone, S. V., Monuteaux, M. C., & Feighner, J. A. (2000). Patterns of alcohol and drug use in adolescents can be predicted by parental substance use disorders. *Pediatrics, 106*(4), 792–797. https://doi.org/10.1542/peds.106.4.792

Blazer, D. G., & Wu, L. (2009). Nonprescription use of pain relievers among middle aged and elderly community adults: National Survey on Drug Use and Health. *Journal of the American Geriatric Society, 57*(7), 1252–1257. https://doi.org/10.1111/j.1532-5415.2009.02306.x

Blow, F., Barry, K., & Galka, A. (2020). Alcohol, prescription, and other drug problems in older adults. In A. J. Herron & T. K. Brennan (Eds.), *The ASAM essentials of addiction medicine* (3rd ed., pp. 233–239). Wolters Kluwer.

Blumenthal, D., & Seervai, S. (2017, October 26). To combat the opioid epidemic, we must be honest about all its causes. *Harvard Business Review.* https://hbr.org/2017/10/to-combat-the-opioid-epidemic-we-must-be-honest-about-all-its-causes

Bobo, L. D., & Thompson, V. (2010). Racialized mass incarceration: Poverty, prejudice, and punishment. In H. R. Markus & P. Moya (Eds.), *Doing race: 21 essays for the 21st century* (pp. 322–355).

Borges, G., Angst, J., Nock, M. K., Ruscio, A. M., Walters, E. E., & Kessler, R. C. (2006). A risk index for 12-month suicide attempts in the National Comorbidity Survey Replication (NCS-R). *Psychological Medicine, 36*(12), 1747–1757.

Brennan, T. K. (2020). Opioid therapy of pain. In A. J. Herron, T. K. Brennan (Eds.), *The ASAM essentials of addiction medicine* (3rd ed., pp. 566–572). Wolters Kluwer.

Briscoe, J., & Cassarett, D. (2018). Medical marijuana use in older adults. *Journal of the American Geriatrics Society, 66*(5), 859–863. https://doi.org/10.1111/jgs.15346

Broyles, L. M., Binswanger, I. A., Jenkins, J. A., Finnell, D. S., Faseru, B., Cavaiola, A., Pugatch, M., & Gordon, A. J. (2014). Confronting inadvertent stigma and pejorative language in addiction scholarship: A recognition and response. *Substance Abuse, 35*(3), 217–221. https://doi.org/10.1080/08897077.2014.930372

Buck, J. A. (2011). The looming expansion and transformation of public substance abuse treatment under the Affordable Care Act. *Health Affairs, 30*(8), 1402–1410. https://doi.org/10.1377/hlthaff.2011.0480

Burda, C. (2020). Substance use disorders: Semantics and stigma. *Nurse Practitioner, 45*(1), 14–17. https://doi.org/10.1097/01.NPR.0000586060.78573.ab

Bush, K., Kivlahan, D. R., McDonell, M. B., Fihn, S. D., & Bradley, K. A. (1998). The AUDIT alcohol consumption questions (AUDIT-C): An effective brief screening test for problem drinking. *Archives of Internal Medicine, 158*(16), 1789–1795. https://doi.org/10.1001/archinte.158.16.1789

Campbell-Heider, N., Finnell, D. S., Feigenbaum, J. C., Feeley, T. H., Rejman, K. S., Austin- Ketch, T., Zulawski, C., & Schmitt, A. (2009). Survey on addictions: Toward curricular change for family nurse practitioners. *International Journal of Nursing Education Scholarship, 6*(1), 1–17. https://pubmed.ncbi.nlm.nih.gov/19222396/

Cano, I., Best, D., Edmonds, M., & Lehman, J. (2017). Recovery capital pathways: Modeling the components of recovery wellbeing. *Drug and Alcohol Abuse, 181*, 11–19. https://www.sciencedirect.com/science/article/abs/pii/S0376871617304830?via%3Dihub

Caplan, G. (1964). *Principles of preventive psychiatry*. Basic Books.

Case, A., & Deaton, A. (2015a). Rising morbidity and mortality in midlife among white non-Hispanic Americans in the 21st century. *Proceedings of the National Academy of Sciences of the United States of America, 112*(49), 15078–81503.

Case, A., & Deaton, A. (2015b). *Suicide, age, and wellbeing: An empirical investigation*. NBER working paper 21279. http://www.nber.org/papers/w21279.pdf

Center for the Application of Prevention Technologies. (n.d.). *Primary, secondary and tertiary prevention strategies & interventions for preventing NMUPD and opioid overdose across the IOM continuum of care*. Substance Abuse and Mental Health Services Administration. https://cadcaworkstation.org/public/DEA360/Shared%20Resources/Root%20Causes%20and%20other%20research/Crosswalk%20PST_USI_models%20with%20NMUPD_PDO__%20examples_9_27_2016_revised.pdf

Center for Substance Abuse Prevention. (2009, January). *Identifying and selecting evidence-based interventions: Revised guidance document for the strategic prevention framework state incentive grant program* (HHS Publication No. [SMA] 09-4205). Substance Abuse and Mental Health Services Administration. https://jjie.org/wp-content/uploads/2018/09/identifying-and-selecting-evidence-based-interventions-samhsa-2009.pdf

Center for Substance Abuse Prevention. (2019, June). *A guide to SAMHSA's Strategic Prevention Framework (SPF)*. Substance Abuse and Mental Health Services Administration. https://www.samhsa.gov/sites/default/files/20190620-samhsa-strategic-prevention-framework-guide.pdf

Center for Substance Abuse Treatment. (2008). An introduction to mutual support groups for alcohol and drug abuse. *Substance Abuse in Brief Fact Sheet, 5*(1). Substance Abuse and Mental Health Services Administration. http://www.william-whitepapers.com/pr/CSAT%20Mutual%20Support%20Groups%202008.pdf

Centers for Disease Control and Prevention. (n.d.). *Alcohol-related disease impact (ARDI)*. https://nccd.cdc.gov/DPH_ARDI/default/default.aspx

Centers for Disease Control and Prevention. (2018a). *Data brief 329: Drug overdose deaths in the United States, 1999–2017.* https://www.cdc.gov/nchs/data/databriefs/db329_tables-508.pdf

Centers for Disease Control and Prevention. (2018b). Suicide rising across the U.S.: More than a mental health concern. *CDC VitalSigns.* https://www.cdc.gov/vitalsigns/pdf/vs-0618-suicide-H.pdf

Centers for Disease Control and Prevention. (2018c). *The opioid crisis: Addressing maternal and infant health.* https://www.cdc.gov/reproductivehealth/maternalinfanthealth/substance-abuse/opioid-use-disorder-pregnancy/index.html

Centers for Disease Control and Prevention. (2019a). *Preventing adverse childhood experiences (ACEs): Leveraging the best available evidence.* https://www.cdc.gov/violenceprevention/pdf/preventingACES.pdf

Centers for Disease Control and Prevention. (2019b, December 10). *Smoking and tobacco use: Youth and tobacco use.* https://www.cdc.gov/tobacco/data_statistics/fact_sheets/youth_data/tobacco_use/index.htm

Centers for Disease Control and Prevention. (2020a, January 3). *Alcohol and public health: Underage drinking.* https://www.cdc.gov/alcohol/fact-sheets/underage-drinking.htm

Centers for Disease Control and Prevention. (2020b, January 21). *PRAMS: Selected 2012 through 2015 maternal and child health (MCH) indicators.* https://www.cdc.gov/prams/prams-data/2019-selected-mch-indicators.html

Centers for Disease Control and Prevention. (2020c, February 25). *Smoking & tobacco use: Outbreak of lung injury associated with the use of e-cigarette, or vaping, products.* https://www.cdc.gov/tobacco/basic_information/e-cigarettes/severe-lung-disease.html

Centers for Disease Control and Prevention. (2020d, March 19). *Drug overdose: Understanding the epidemic.* https://www.cdc.gov/drugoverdose/epidemic/index.html

Centers for Disease Control and Prevention. (2020e, April 28). *Smoking & tobacco use: Smoking during pregnancy.* https://www.cdc.gov/tobacco/basic_information/health_effects/pregnancy/index.htm

Centers for Disease Control and Prevention. (2020f, April 30). *Fetal alcohol spectrum disorders (FASDs): Alcohol use in pregnancy.* https://www.cdc.gov/ncbddd/fasd/alcohol-use.html

Centers for Disease Control and Prevention. (2020g, June 10). *HIV: HIV in the United States and dependent areas.* https://www.cdc.gov/hiv/statistics/overview/ataglance.html

Centers for Disease Control and Prevention. (2021, January 26). *Opioids: Commonly used terms.* https://www.cdc.gov/opioids/basics/terms.html

Centers for Medicare and Medicaid Services. (n.d.). *Essential health benefits standards: Ensuring quality, affordable coverage.* https://www.cms.gov/CCIIO/Resources/Fact-Sheets-and-FAQs/ehb-2-20-2013

Centers for Medicare and Medicaid Services. (2014, January). *Partners in integrity: What is the prescriber's role in preventing the diversion of prescription drugs?* https://www.pharmacy.umn.edu/sites/pharmacy.umn.edu/files/prescriber_role_in_preventing_diversion.pdf

Chariyeva, Z., Golin, C. E., Earp, J. A., Maman, S., Suchindran, C., & Zimmer, C. (2013). The role of self-efficacy and motivation to explain the effect of motivational interviewing time on changes in risky sexual behavior among people living with HIV: a mediation analysis. *AIDS and Behavior, 17*(2), 813–823.

Chisholm, B. (1951). *Outline for a study group on world health and the survival of the human race: Material drawn from articles and speeches.* Geneva: World Health Organization. https://apps.who.int/iris/handle/10665/330666

Clancy, C., & Fornili, K. (2019). International Nurses Society on Addictions: Strategic plan for global development to shape policy and strengthen nursing influence. *Journal of Addictions Nursing, 30*(3), 226–231. https://doi.org/10.1097/JAN.0000000000000299

Clancy, C., Oyefeso, A., & Ghodse, H. (2007). Role development and career stages in addiction nursing: An exploratory study. *Journal of Advanced Nursing, 57*(2), 161–171. https://doi.org/10.1111/j.1365-2648.2006.04088.x

Community Anti-Drug Coalitions of America. (n.d.). *The comprehensive addiction and recovery act (CARA).* https://www.cadca.org/comprehensive-addiction-and-recovery-act-cara

Confidentiality of Records, 42 U.S.C. § 290dd-2 (2010).

Confidentiality of Substance Use Disorder Patient Records, 42 C.F.R. §§ 2.1–2.4, §§ 2.11–2.23, §§ 2.31–2.35, §§ 2.51–2.53, §§ 2.61–2.67. (2017).

Corey, G., Corey, M. S., & Corey, C. (2018). *Issues and ethics in the helping professions* (10th ed.). Boston, MA: Cengage Learning.

Corrigan, P. W., Schomerus, G., Shuman, V., Kraus, D., Perlick, D., Harnish, A., Kulesza, M., Kane-Willis, K., Qin, S., & Smelson, D. (2017). Developing a research agenda for reducing the stigma of addictions, Part I: Lessons from the mental health stigma literature. *American Journal on Addictions, 26*(1), 67–74. https://doi.org/10.1111/ajad.12458

Cross, T. L., Bazron, B. J., Dennis, K. W., & Isaacs, M. R. (1989). *Towards a culturally competent system of care: A monograph on effective services for minority children who are severely emotionally disturbed.* Washington, DC: Georgetown University Child Development Center, CASSP Technical Assistance Center. https://files.eric.ed.gov/fulltext/ED330171.pdf

Crothers, C. E., & Dorrian, J. (2011). Determinants of nurses' attitudes toward the care of patients with alcohol problems. *ISRN Nursing, 2011,* 1–11. https://doi.org/10.5402/2011/821514

Davis, A. (2017). Introduction. In A. Davis (Ed.), Policing the black man: Arrest, prosecution, and imprisonment (pp. xi–xxiv). New York, NY: Pantheon Books.

Dennis, M. L., Scott, C. K., Funk, R., & Foss, M. A. (2005). The duration and correlates of addiction and treatment careers. *Journal of Substance Abuse Treatment, 28*(2), S51–S62. https://doi.org/10.1016/j.jsat.2004.10.013

Dey, J., Rosenoff, E., West, K., Ali, M. M., McClellan, C., Mutter, R., Patton, L., Teich, J., & Woodward, A. (2016). *ASPE issue brief: Benefits of Medicaid expansion for behavioral health.* U.S. Department of Health and Human Services, Office of the Assistant Secretary for Planning and Evaluation. https://aspe.hhs.gov/system/files/pdf/190506/BHMedicaidExpansion.pdf

DiClemente, C. (2006). *Addiction and change: How addictions develop and addicted people recover.* Guilford Press.

Donovan, D. M., & Floyd, A. S. (2008). Facilitating involvement in twelve-step programs. *Recent Developments in Alcoholism,* 18, 303–320. https://doi.org/10.1007/978-0-387-77725-2_17

Douaihy, A., Dailey, D., Marlatt, G. A., & Donovan, D. (2020) Relapse prevention clinical models and intervention strategies. In A. J. Herron & T. K. Brennan (Eds.), *The ASAM essentials of addiction medicine* (3rd ed., pp. 402–407). Wolters Kluwer.

Dudley J. (2000). Confronting stigma within the services system. *Social Work, 45*(5), 449–455. https://doi.org/10.1093/sw/45.5.449.

DuPont, R. L., McLellan, A. T., White, W. L., Merlo, L. J., & Gold, M. S. (2009). Setting the standard for recovery: Physicians' health programs. *Journal of Substance Abuse Treatment, 36*(2), 159–171. https://doi.org/10.1016/j.jsat.2008.01.004

Dyer, J. (2000). The perpetual prison machine: How America profits from crime. Boulder, CO: Westview Press.

European Monitoring Centre for Drugs and Drug Addiction. (2016). *Best practice portal.* http://www.emcdda.europa.eu/best-practice

Farokhzadian, J., Khajouei, R., & Ahmadian, L. (2015). Evaluating factors associated with implementing evidence-based practice in nursing. *Journal of Evaluation in Clinical Practice, 21*(6), 1107–1113. https://doi.org/10.1111/jep.12480

Finnell, D., Savage, C., Hansen, B., Sanchez, M., White, K., Johnson, J., & Seale, J. (2018). Integrating substance use content in an "overcrowded" nursing curriculum. *Nurse Educator, 43*(3), 128–131. https://doi.org/10.1097/NNE.0000000000000438

Fogger, S., & Dobbs, G. (2020). Treating pain while mindful of opioid risks. *American Nurse Today.* https://www.myamericannurse.com/treating-pain-while-mindful-of-opioid-risks/

Ford, J. D. (2013). *Treatment of complex trauma: A sequenced, relationship-based approach.* Guilford Press.

Fornili, K. (2016a). Part 1: The theoretical basis for recovery-oriented management of substance use disorders in primary care. *Journal of Addictions Nursing, 27*(2), 78–85. https://doi.org/10.1097/JAN.0000000000000118

Fornili, K. (2016b). Part 2: Screening, brief intervention and referral to treatment plus recovery management. *Journal of Addictions Nursing, 27*(2), 86–93. https://doi.org/10.1097/JAN.0000000000000119

Fornili, K. (2017). Socialized risk and privatized profit: What addictions nurses need to know about the potential repeal of the Affordable Care Act. *Journal of Addictions Nursing, 28*(3), 157–165. https://doi.org/10.1097/JAN.0000000000000184

Fornili, K. (2018). Racialized mass incarceration and the war on drugs: A critical race theory appraisal. *Journal of Addiction Nursing, 29*(1), 65–72. https://doi.org/10.1097/JAN.0000000000000215

Fouladi, F., Mitchell, J., Cosby, R., Engel, S., Crow, S., Hill, L., Le George, D., Power, P., & Steffen, K. (2015, November 23). Prevalence of alcohol and other substances use in patients with eating disorders. *European Eating Disorders Review, 23*(6), 531–536. https://doi.org/10.1002/erv.2410

Fowler, M. (2015). *Guide to the code of ethics for nurses with interpretive statements: Development, interpretation, and application* (2nd ed.). Silver Spring, MD: American Nurses Association.

Fox, A. D., Maradiaga, J., Weiss, L., Sanchez, J., Starrels, J. L., & Cunningham, C. O. (2015). Release from incarceration, relapse to opioid use and the potential for buprenorphine maintenance treatment: A qualitative study of the perceptions of former inmates with opioid use disorder. *Addiction Science and Clinical Practice, 10*(1), 1–9. https://doi.org/10.1186/s13722-014-0023-0

Fraser, S. (2016). Articulating addiction in alcohol and other drug policy: A multiverse of habits. *International Journal of Drug Policy, 31*, 6–14. https://doi.org/10.1016/j.drugpo.2015.10.014

Garbin, M. (2019a). *Executive summary for the Addictions Nursing Certification Board: Practice analysis/role delineation of addictions advanced practice nursing (CARN-AP).* Center for Nursing Education and Testing. https://www.intnsa.org/wp-content/uploads/ancb/carnap2018.pdf

Garbin, M. (2019b). *Executive summary for the Addictions Nursing Certification Board: Practice analysis/role delineation of addictions nursing (CARN).* Center for Nursing Education and Testing. https://www.intnsa.org/wp-content/uploads/ancb/carn2018.pdf

Garland, D. W. (Ed.). (2001). *Mass imprisonment: Social causes and consequences.* Sage.

Garnick, D. W., Lee, M. T., Horgan, C. M., & Acevedo, A. (2009). Adapting Washington Circle performance measures for public sector substance abuse treatment systems. *Journal of Substance Abuse Treatment, 36*(3), 265–277.

Ghosh, T. S., Vigil, D. I., Maffey, A., Tolliver, R., Van Dyke, M., Kattari, L., Krug, H., Reed, J. K., & Wolk, L. (2017). Lessons learned after three years of legalized, recreational cannabis: The Colorado experience. *Preventive Medicine, 104*, 4–6. https://doi.org/10.1016/j.ypmed.2017.02.021

Goffman E. (1963). *Stigma: Notes on the management of spoiled identity.* Prentice Hall.

Goldberger, B. A., Maxwell, J. C., Campbell, A., & Wilford, B. B. (2013). Uniform standards and case definitions for classifying opioid-related deaths: Recommendations by a SAMHSA consensus panel. *Journal of Addictive Diseases, 32*(3), 231–243. https://doi.org/10.1080/10550887.2013.824334

Gordon R. (1983). An operational classification of disease prevention. *Public Health Reports, 98*(2), 107–109. https://www.ncbi.nlm.nih.gov/pmc/articles/PMC1424415/

Green, J. (2006). Banking on the prison boom. In T. Herivel & P. Wright (Eds.), Prison profiteers: Who makes money from mass incarceration (pp. 3Y26).

Green, K. E., & Feinstein, B. A. (2012). Substance use in lesbian, gay, and bisexual populations: An update on empirical research and implications for treatment. *Psychology of Addictive Behaviors, 26*(2), 265–278. https://doi.org/10.1037/a0025424

Grossman, E., Benjamin-Neelone, S., & Sonnenscheim, S. (2020). Alcohol consumption during the COVID-19 pandemic: A cross-sectional survey of U.S. adults. *International Journal of Environmental Research and Public Health, 17*, 9189. https://doi.org/10.3390/ijerph17249189

Guyer, J., & Scott, K. (2020, May 2). State strategies for helping individuals with opioid use disorder through the COVID-19 epidemic. *Health Affairs Blog.* https://www.healthaffairs.org/do/10.1377/forefront.20200429.476954

Haight, S. C., Ko, J. Y., Tong, V. T., Bohm, M. K., & Callaghan, W. M. (2018). Opioid use disorder documented at delivery hospitalization—United States, 1999–2014. *Morbidity Mortality Weekly Report, 67*(31), 845–849. https://doi.org/10.15585/mmwr.mm6731a1

Harris, M., & Fallot, R. D. (2001). *Using trauma theory to design service systems.* Jossey-Bass/Wiley.

Hawk, M., Coulter, R., Egan, J., Fisk, S., Friedman, M., Tula, M., & Kinsky, S. (2017). Harm reduction principles for healthcare settings. *Harm Reduction Journal, 14*(1), 1–9. https://doi.org/10.1186/s12954-017-0196-4

Health Insurance Portability and Accountability Act. Pub. L. No. 104–191, § 264, 110 Stat. 1936 (1996).

Heather, N., Smailes, D., & Cassidy, P. (2008). Development of a readiness ruler for use with alcohol brief interventions. *Drug and Alcohol Dependence, 98*(3), 235–240. https://doi.org/10.1016/j.drugalcdep.2008.06.005

Hendershot, C. S., Witkiewitz, K., George, W. H., & Marlatt, G. A. (2011). Relapse prevention for addictive behaviors. *Substance Abuse Treatment, Prevention, & Policy, 6*(1), 1–17. https://doi.org/10.1186/1747-597X-6-17

Hser, Y. I., Evans, E., Huang, D., & Anglin, D. M. (2014). Relationship between drug treatment services, retention, and outcomes. *Psychiatric Services, 55*(7), 767–774. doi.org/10.1176/appi.ps.55.7.767

Hook, J., Davis, D., Owen, J., Worthington, E., & Utsey, S. (2013). Cultural humility: Measuring openness to culturally diverse clients. *Journal of Counseling Psychology, 60*(3). 353–366. https://doi.org/10.1037/a0032595

Humphreys, K. (2004). *Circles of recovery: Self-help organizations for addictions.* University Press.

Institute for Research, Education & Training in Addictions. (n.d.). *Addiction glossary.* https://ireta.org/about-addiction/glossary

Institute of Medicine. (1990). *Broadening the base of treatment for alcohol problems: Report of a study by the Institute of Medicine Division of Mental Health and Behavioral Medicine.* National Academies Press.

Institute of Medicine. (2001). *Crossing the quality chasm: A new health system for the 21st century.* National Academies Press.

Institute of Medicine. (2006). *Improving the quality of health care for mental and substance-use conditions: Quality chasm series.* National Academies Press.

Institute of Medicine. (2011). *The future of nursing: Leading change, advancing health.* National Academies Press.

International Association for the Study of Pain. (n.d.). *Pain in older persons.* https://www.iasp-pain.org/GlobalYear/PaininOlderPersons

International Association for the Study of Pain. (2020, July 16). *IASP announces revised definition of pain.* https://www.iasp-pain.org/publications/iasp-news/iasp-announces-revised-definition-of-pain/

International Council of Nurses. (2002). *Nursing definitions.* https://www.icn.ch/nursing-policy/nursing-definitions

International Council of Nurses. (2012). *The ICN code of ethics for nurses.* https://www.icn.ch/sites/default/files/inline-files/2012_ICN_Codeofethicsfornurses_%20eng.pdf

International Council of Nurses. (2013). *Cultural and linguistic competence: ICN position statement.* https://www.icn.ch/sites/default/files/inline-files/B03_Cultural_Linguistic_Competence.pdf

Joanna Briggs Institute. (2018). *The Joanna Briggs Institute.* http://joannabriggs.org.

Johnston, L. D., Miech, R. A., O'Malley, P. M., Bachman, J. G., Schulenberg, J. E., & Patrick, M. E. (2019). *Monitoring the Future national survey results on drug use 1975–2018: Overview, key findings on adolescent drug use.* Ann Arbor: Institute for Social Research, University of Michigan.

The Joint Commission. (2014). *Substance use.* https://www.jointcommission.org/measurement/measures/substance-use/

Kaiser Family Foundation. (2017). Most Americans say federal and state governments are not doing enough to combat prescription painkiller and heroin abuse; large majorities believe a wide range of strategies would be effective. *KFF newsroom.* https://www.kff.org/health-reform/press-release/most-americans-say-federal-and-state-governments-are-not-doing-enough-to-combat-prescription-painkiller-and-heroin-abuse-large-majorities-believe-wide-range-of-strategies-would-be-effective/

Kaiser Family Foundation. (2020, May 29). *Status of state Medicaid expansion decisions: Interactive map.* https://www.kff.org/medicaid/issue-brief/status-of-state-medicaid-expansion-decisions-interactive-map/#

Kamer, R. S., Warshafsky, S., & Kamer, G. C. (2020). Change in traffic fatality rates in the first 4 states to legalize recreational marijuana. *JAMA Internal Medicine, 180*(8), 1119–1120. https://doi.org/10.1001/jamainternmed.2020.1769

Kann, L., McManus, T., Harris, W. A., Shanklin, S. L., Flint, K. H., Queen, B., Lowry, R., Chyen, D., Whittle, L., Thornton, J., Lim, C., Bradford, D., Yamakawa, Y., Leon, M., Brener, B., & Ethier, K. A. (2018). Youth risk behavior surveillance—United States, 2017. *CDC Morbidity and Mortality Weekly Report, 67*(8). https://www.cdc.gov/healthyyouth/data/yrbs/pdf/2017/ss6708.pdf

Kelly, J. F., Saitz, R., Wakeman, S. (2016). Language, substance use disorders, and policy: The need to reach consensus on an "addiction-ary." *Alcoholism Treatment Quarterly, 34*(1), 116–123. https://doi.org/10.1080/07347324.2016.1113103

Kelly, J. F., Stout, R. L., Magill, M., Tonigan, J. S., & Pagano, M. E. (2011). Spirituality in recovery: A lagged mediational analysis of Alcoholics Anonymous' principal theoretical mechanism of behavior change. *Alcoholism: Clinical & Experimental Research, 35*(3), 454–463. https://doi.org/10.1111/j.1530-0277.2010.01362.x

Kelly, P., Vottero, B., & Christie-McCauliffe, C. (2018). *Introduction to quality and safety education for nurses: Core competencies for nursing leadership and management* (2nd ed.). Springer Publishing Company.

Kerr, W. C., Lui, C., & Ye, Y. (2017). Trends and age, period and cohort effects for marijuana use prevalence in the 1984–2015 US National Alcohol Surveys. *Addiction, 113*, 473–481. https://doi.org/10.1111/add.14031

Koivunen, M., Välimäki, M., & Hätönen, H. (2010). Nurses' information retrieval skills in psychiatric hospitals—Are the requirements for evidence-based practice fulfilled? *Nurse Education in Practice, 10*(1), 27–31. https://doi.org/10.1016/j.nepr.2009.03.004

Kochanek, K. D., Murphy, S., Xu, J., & Arias, E. (2017). Mortality in the United States, 2016. *National Center for Health Statistics Data Brief, 293.* https://www.cdc.gov/nchs/data/databriefs/db293.pdf

Kunyk, D. (2015). Substance use disorders among registered nurses: Prevalence, risks and perceptions in a disciplinary jurisdiction. *Journal of Nursing Management, 23*(1), 54–64.

Kurti, A., Keith, D., Noble, B., Priest, J., Sprague, B., & Higgins, S. (2016). Characterizing the intersection of co-occurring risk factors for illicit drug abuse and dependence in a U.S. nationally representative sample. *Preventive Medicine, 92,* 118–125. https://doi.org/10.1016/j.ypmed.2016.09.030

Legal Action Center. (2009). *Know your rights: Rights for individuals on medication-assisted treatment* (HHS Publication No. [SMA] 09-4449). Rockville, MD: Center for Substance Abuse Treatment, Substance Abuse and Mental Health Services Administration. https://atforum.com/documents/Know_Your_Rights_Brochure_0110.pdf

Lipari, R. N., & Van Horn, S. L. (2017, August 24). *Children living with parents who have a substance use disorder: The CBHSQ Report.* Center for Behavioral Health Statistics and Quality, Substance Abuse and Mental Health Services Administration. https://www.samhsa.gov/data/sites/default/files/report_3223/ShortReport-3223.pdf

MacAfee, L. K., Dalton, V., & Terplan, M. (2019). Pregnancy intention, risk perception, and contraceptive use in pregnant women who use drugs. *Journal of Addiction Medicine, 13*(3), 177–181. https://doi.org/10.1097/ADM.0000000000000471

Mahmoud, K. F., Finnell, D., Savage, C. L., Puskar, K. R., & Mitchell, A. M. (2017). A concept analysis of substance misuse to inform contemporary terminology. *Archives of Psychiatric Nursing, 31*(6), 532–540. https://doi.org/10.1016/j.apnu.2017.06.004

Mahmoud, K. F., Finnell, D., Lindsay, D., MacFarland, C., Marze, H., Scolieri, B. B., & Mitchell, A. M. (2018). Can screening, brief intervention and referral to treatment education and clinical exposure impact nursing students' stigma toward alcohol and opioid use? *Journal of the American Psychiatric Nurses Association, 25*(6), 467–475. https://doi.org/10.1177/1078390318811570

Malone, D. T., Hill, M. N., & Rubino, T. (2010). Adolescent cannabis use and psychosis: Epidemiology and neurodevelopmental models. *British Journal of Pharmacology, 160*(3), 511–522. https://doi.org/10.1111/j.1476-5381.2010.00721.x

Marcus, M. T., Savage, C., & Finnell, D. S. (2020). Nursing roles in addressing addiction. In A. J. Herron & T. K. Brennan (Eds.), *The ASAM principles of addiction medicine* (5th ed.). Lippincott Williams & Wilkins.

Marion, L., Douglas, M., Lavin, M. A., Barr, N., Gazaway, S., Thomas, E., & Bickford, C. (2017). Implementing the new ANA standard 8: Culturally congruent practice. *Online Journal of Issues in Nursing, 22*(1). https://ojin.nursingworld.org/MainMenuCategories/ANAMarketplace/ANAPeriodicals/OJIN/TableofContents/Vol-22-2017/No1-Jan-2017/Articles-Previous-Topics/Implementing-the-New-ANA-Standard-8.html

Marlatt, G. A. (1985). Relapse prevention: Theoretical rationale and overview of the model. In G. A. Marlatt and J. R. Gordon (Eds.), *Relapse prevention* (pp. 3–70). Guilford Press.

Mattson, M., Lipari, R. N., Hays, C., & Van Horn, S. L. (2017). A day in the life of older adults: Substance use facts. *CBHSQ Report.* Center for Behavioral Health Statistics and Quality, Substance Abuse and Mental Health Services Administration.

Mauer, M. (2011). Addressing racial disparities in incarceration. *Prison Journal*, *91*(3 Suppl.), 87S–101S. https://doi.org/10.1177/0032885511415227

McLellan, A. T., Lewis, C., O'Brien, C. P., & Kleber, H. (2000). Drug dependence, a chronic medical illness: Implications for treatment, insurance, and outcomes evaluation. *Journal of the American Medical Association*, *284*(13), 1689–1695. https://doi.org/10.1001/jama.284.13.1689

McLellan, A. T., Skipper, G. S., Campbell, M., & DuPont, R. L. (2008). Five-year outcomes in a cohort study of physicians treated for substance use disorders in the United States. *British Journal of Medicine*, *337*, a2038. https://doi.org/10.1136/bmj.a2038

Medley, G., Lipari, R., Bose, J., Cribb, D., Kroutil, L., & McHenry, G. (2016, October). Sexual orientation and estimates of adult substance use and mental health: Results from the 2015 National Survey on Drug Use and Health. *NSDUH Data Review*. Substance Abuse and Mental Health Services Administration. https://www.samhsa.gov/data/sites/default/files/NSDUH-SexualOrientation-2015/NSDUH-SexualOrientation-2015/NSDUH-SexualOrientation-2015.pdf

Mee-Lee, D., & Shulman, G. D. (2020). The ASAM criteria and matching patients to treatment. In A. J. Herron & T. K. Brennan (Eds.), *The ASAM essentials of addiction medicine* (3rd ed., pp. 172–178). Wolters Kluwer.

Mee-Lee, D., Shulman, G., Fishman, J., Gastfried, D., & Miller, M. (eds.). (2013). *The ASAM criteria: Treatment for addictive, substance-related, and co-occurring conditions* (3rd ed.). American Society of Addiction Medicine.

Melnyk, B. M., & Fineout-Overholt, E. (2005). *Evidence-based practice in nursing & healthcare: A guide to best practice.* Lippincott Williams & Wilkins.

Melnyk, B. M., Fineout-Overholt, E., Stillwell, S. B., & Williamson, K. M. (2010). Evidence-based practice: Step by step: The seven steps of evidence-based practice. *American Journal of Nursing*, *110*(1), 51–53. https://doi.org/10.1097/01.NAJ.0000366056.06605.d2

Miller, J. (2013, November 7). *The waterfall effect: Transformative impacts of the ACA coverage expansions and systems reforms for people with mental health conditions.* Carter Center. https://www.cartercenter.org/resources/pdfs/health/mental_health/symposium/2013/joel-miller.pdf

Miller, W. R., & Rollnick, S. (1991). *Motivational interviewing: Preparing people to change addictive behavior.* Guilford Press.

Miller, W. R., & Rollnick, S. (2013). *Motivational interviewing: Helping people change* (3rd ed.). Guilford Press.

Minkoff, K., & Covell, N. (2019, August). *Integrated systems and services for people with co-occurring mental health and substance use conditions: What's known, what's new, and what's now?* https://www.nasmhpd.org/sites/default/files/TAC_Paper_8_508C.pdf

Mollica, M. A., Hyman, Z., & Mann, C. M. (2011). Alcohol-related content in undergraduate nursing curricula in the northeastern United States. *Journal of Psychosocial Nursing, 49*(6), 22–31. https://doi.org/10.3928/02793695-20110503-01

Monroe, T., Kenaga, H., Dietrich, M. S., Carter, M. A., & Cowan, R. L. (2013). The prevalence of employed nurses identified or enrolled in substance use monitoring programs. *Nursing Research, 62*(1), 10–15. https://doi.org/10.1097/NNR.0b013e31826ba3ca

Monroe, T., Pearson, F., & Kenaga, H. (2008). Procedures for handling cases of substance abuse among nurses: A comparison of disciplinary and alternative programs. *Journal of Addictions Nursing, 19*(3), 156–161. https://doi.org/10.1080/10884600802306024

Moon, M. W., Fornili, K., & O'Briant, A. L. (2007). Risk comparison among youth who report sex with same-sex versus both-sex partners. *Youth & Society, 38*(3), 267–284. https://doi.org/10.1177/0044118X06287689

Moyer, V. A., & the U.S. Preventive Services Task Force. (2013). Screening and behavioral counseling interventions in primary care to reduce alcohol misuse: U.S. Preventive Services Task Force recommendation statement. *Annals of Internal Medicine, 159*(3), 210–218. https://doi.org/10.7326/0003-4819-159-3-201308060-00652

Nagel, M., & Fougere, M. A. (2017). Nursing roles in care of patients with substance use disorder. *Journal of Addiction Nursing, 28*(3), 109. https://doi.org/10.1097/JAN.0000000000000183

Nash, A. J., Marcus, M. T., Cron, S., Scamp, N., Truitt, M., McKenna, Z. (2017). Preparing nursing students to work with patients with alcohol or drug-related problems. *Journal of Addictions Nursing, 28*(3), 124–130. https://doi.org/10.1097/JAN.0000000000000175

National Academies of Sciences, Engineering, and Medicine. (2017, January 12). *The health effects of cannabis and cannabinoids: The current state of evidence and recommendations for research.* National Academies Press. https://doi.org/10.17226/24625

National Academies of Sciences, Engineering, and Medicine. (2021). *The future of nursing 2020–2030: Charting a path to achieve health equity.* National Academies Press. https://doi.org/10.17226/25982.

National Center for Chronic Disease Prevention and Health Promotion Office on Smoking and Health. (2014). *The health consequences of smoking—50 years of progress: A report of the Surgeon General.* U.S. Department of Health and Human Services, Centers for Disease Control and Prevention. https://pubmed.ncbi.nlm.nih.gov/24455788/

National Council for Behavioral Health. (2017). *Unite4BH.* https://www.thenationalcouncil.org/policy-action/unite4bh

National Council of State Boards of Nursing. (2008, July 7). *Consensus model for APRNs regulation: Licensure, accreditation, certification & education.* https://www.ncsbn.org/Consensus_Model_Report.pdf

National Institute on Alcohol Abuse and Alcoholism. (n.d.). *Drinking levels defined.* https://www.niaaa.nih.gov/alcohol-health/overview-alcohol-consumption/moderate-binge-drinking

National Institute on Alcohol Abuse and Alcoholism. (2007). *Helping patients who drink too much: A clinician's guide* (NIH Publication No. 07–3769). https://pubs.niaaa.nih.gov/publications/Practitioner/CliniciansGuide2005/guide.pdf

National Institute on Alcohol Abuse and Alcoholism. (2008, July). Alcohol and other drugs. *Alcohol Alert, 76,* 1–6. https://pubs.niaaa.nih.gov/publications/aa76/AA76.pdf

National Institute on Alcohol Abuse and Alcoholism. (2019, December). *Medications development program.* https://www.niaaa.nih.gov/medications-development-program

National Institute on Drug Abuse. (n.d.). *Substance use and SUDs in LGBTQ* populations.* https://www.drugabuse.gov/drug-topics/substance-use-suds-in-lgbtq-populations

National Institutes on Drug Abuse. (2014, April 18). *Principles of drug abuse treatment for criminal justice populations—A research-based guide.* https://www.drugabuse.gov/publications/principles-drug-abuse-treatment-criminal-justice-populations-research-based-guide

National Institute on Drug Abuse. (2017, October 25). *Addressing the opioid crisis means confronting socioeconomic disparities.* https://www.drugabuse.gov/about-nida/noras-blog/2017/10/addressing-opioid-crisis-means-confronting-socioeconomic-disparities

National Institute on Drug Abuse. (2018a, January). *Principles of drug addiction treatment: A research-based guide* (3rd ed.). https://www.drugabuse.gov/publications/principles-drug-addiction-treatment-research-based-guide-third-edition/principles-effective-treatment

National Institute on Drug Abuse. (2018b, May 31). *Cigarette smoking increases the likelihood of drug use relapse.* https://www.drugabuse.gov/news-events/nida-notes/2018/05/cigarette-smoking-increases-likelihood-drug-use-relapse

National Institute on Drug Abuse. (2018c, July 2). *Media guide.* https://archives.drugabuse.gov/publications/media-guide

National Institute on Drug Abuse. (2019, April). *Marijuana research report: Is marijuana addictive?* https://www.drugabuse.gov/publications/research-reports/marijuana/marijuana-addictive

National Institute on Drug Abuse. (2020a, April 1). *Marijuana potency.* https://www.drugabuse.gov/drugs-abuse/marijuana/marijuana-potency

National Institute on Drug Abuse. (2020b, May 27). *Opioid overdose crisis.* https://www.drugabuse.gov/drug-topics/opioids/opioid-overdose-crisis

National Institutes on Drug Abuse. (2020c, June). *Criminal justice drugfacts.* https://www.drugabuse.gov/publications/drugfacts/criminal-justice

National Institute on Drug Abuse. (2020d, July). *Marijuana research report.* https://www.drugabuse.gov/download/1380/marijuana-research-report.pdf?v=d9e67cbd412ae5f340206c1a0d9c2bfd

National Quality Forum. (2014). *NQF endorses behavioral health measures* [Press release]. https://www.qualityforum.org/News_And_Resources/Press_Releases/2014/NQF_Endorses_Behavioral_Health_Measures.aspx

North Carolina Board of Nursing & North Carolina State Opioid Treatment Authority. (2021). *Joint position statement.* https://www.ncbon.com/vdownloads/position-statements-decision-trees/opioid-treatment-programs.pdf

O'Connell, M., Boat, T., & Warner, K. (Eds.). (2009). *Preventing mental, emotional, and behavioral disorders among young people: Progress and possibilities.* National Academies Press.

Office of the Assistant Secretary for Planning and Evaluation. (2016, March 28). *Benefits of Medicaid expansion for behavioral health.* U.S. Department of Health and Human Services. https://aspe.hhs.gov/system/files/pdf/190506/BHMedicaidExpansion.pdf

Office of the Assistant Secretary for Planning and Evaluation. (2017, January 11). *Continuing progress on the opioid epidemic: The role of the Affordable Care Act.* U.S. Department of Health and Human Services. https://aspe.hhs.gov/system/files/pdf/255456/ACAOpioid.pdf

Office of Disease Prevention and Health Promotion. (2019). *Healthy People 2030: What is the Healthy People 2030 framework?* https://www.healthypeople.gov/2020/About-Healthy-People/Development-Healthy-People-2030/Framework

Office of Minority Health. (2013). *National standards for culturally and linguistically appropriate services (CLAS) in health and health care.* Washington, DC: U.S. Department of Health and Human Services. https://thinkculturalhealth.hhs.gov/assets/pdfs/EnhancedNationalCLASStandards.pdf

Orgera, K., & Tolbert, J. (2019). *Key facts about uninsured adults with opioid addiction.* https://www.kff.org/uninsured/issue-brief/key-facts-about-uninsured-adults-with-opioid-use-disorder/

Oquendo, M. A., & Volkow, N. D. (2018). Suicide: A silent contributor to opioid-overdose deaths. *New England Journal of Medicine, 378*(17), 1567–1569. https://doi.org/10.1056/NEJMp1801417

Owens, P. L., Barrett, M. L., Weiss, A. J., Washington, R. E., & Kronick, R. (2014, August). *Hospital inpatient utilization related to opioid overuse among adults, 1993–2012* (Statistical brief #177). Agency for Healthcare Research and Quality. https://www.hcup-us.ahrq.gov/reports/statbriefs/sb177-Hospitalizations-for-Opioid-Overuse.pdf

Paradise, J. (2017, March). *Issue brief: Restructuring Medicaid in the American Health Care Act: Five key considerations.* http://files.kff.org/attachment/Issue-Brief-Restructuring-Medicaid-in-the-American-Health-Care-Act

Park-Lee, E., Lipari, R., Hedden, S., Kroutil, L., & Porter, J. (2017, September). Receipt of services for substance use and mental health issues among adults: Results from the 2016 National Survey on Drug Use and Health. *CBHSQ Data Review.* Substance Abuse and Mental Health Services Administration. https://www.samhsa.gov/data/sites/default/files/NSDUH-DR-FFR2-2016/NSDUH-DR-FFR2-2016.htm

Patel, K. V., Guralnik, J. M., Dansie, E. J., & Turk, D. C. (2014). Prevalence and impact of pain among older adults in the United States: Findings from the 2011 National Health and Aging Trends Study. *Pain, 154*(12), 2649–2657. https://doi.org/10.1016/j.pain.2013.07.029

Patient Protection and Affordable Care Act, 42 U.S.C. § 18001 *et seq.* (2010).

Paul Wellstone and Pete Domenici Mental Health Parity and Addiction Equity Act of 2008 (MHPAEA), H.R. 6983, 110th Cong. (2008).

Peleg-Oren, N., & Teichman, M. (2006). Young children of parents with substance use disorders (SUD): A review of the literature and implications for social work practice. *Journal of Social Work Practice in the Addictions, 6*(1–2), 49–61. https://doi.org/10.1300/J160v06n01_03

Polen, M. R., Whitlock, E. P., Wisdom, J. P., Nygren, P., & Bougatsos, C. (2008). *Screening in primary care settings for illicit drug use: Staged systematic review for the United States Preventive Services Task Force.* Rockville, MD: Agency for Healthcare Research and Quality. https://www.ncbi.nlm.nih.gov/books/NBK33960/

Poznyak, V., Saraceno, B., & Obot, I. (2005). Breaking the vicious cycle of determinants and consequences of alcohol use. *Bulletin of the World Health Organization, 83*(11), 801–880. https://www.who.int/bulletin/volumes/83/11/editorial21105html/en/

Prochaska, J., & DeClemente, C. (1982). Transtheoretical therapy: Toward a more integrative model of change. *Psychotherapy Therapy & Practice, 19*(3), 276–288. https://doi.org/10.1037/h0088437

Qureshi, R., Zha, P., Kim, S., & Hindin, P., Naqvi, Z., Holly, C., Dubbs, W., & Ritch, W. (2017). Health care needs and care utilization among lesbian, gay, bisexual, and transgender populations in New Jersey. *Journal of Homosexuality, 65*(2), 167–180. https://doi.org/10.1080/00918369.2017.1311555

Rahm, A. K., Boggs, J. M., Martin, C., Price, D. W., Beck, A., Backer, T. E., & Dearing, J. W. (2015). Facilitators and barriers to implementing screening, brief intervention, and referral to treatment (SBIRT) in primary care in integrated health care settings. *Substance Abuse, 36*(3), 281–288. https://doi.org/10.1080/08897077.2014.951140

Reinholdz, H., Fornazar, R., Bendtsen, P., & Spak, F. (2013). Comparison of systematic versus targeted screening for detection of risky drinking in primary care. *Alcohol and Alcoholism, 48*(2), 172–179. http://doi.org/10.1093/alcalc/ags137

Reisfield, G., Bertholf, R., Goldberger, B., & Dupont, R. (2020). Practical considerations for drug testing. In A. J. Herron & T. K. Brennan (Eds.), *The ASAM essentials of addiction medicine* (3rd ed., pp. 659–666). Wolters Kluwer.

Reisner, S. L., Biello, K., Hughto, J. M., Kuhns, L., Mayer, K. H., Garofalo, R., & Mimiagoa, M. J. (2016). Psychiatric diagnoses and comorbidities in a diverse multicity cohort of young transgender women: Baseline findings from Project LifeSkills. *JAMA Pediatrics*, *170*(5), 481–486. https://doi.org/10.1001/jamapediatrics. 2016.0067

Reisner, S. L., Jadwin-Cakmak, L., White Hughto, J. M., Martinez, M., Salomon, L., & Harper, G. W. (2017). Characterizing the HIV prevention and care continua in a sample of transgender youth in the U.S. *AIDS and Behavior*, *21*(12), 3312–3327. https://doi.org/10.1007/s10461-017-1938-8

Renstrom, M., Ferri, M., & Mandil, A. (2017). Substance use prevention: Evidence-based intervention. *Eastern Mediterranean Health Journal*, *23*(3), 198–205. http://www.emro.who.int/emhj-volume-23-2017/volume-23-issue-3/substance-use-prevention-evidence-based-intervention.html

Riner, M. E. (2015). Using implementation science as the core of the doctor of nursing practice inquiry project. *Journal of Professional Nursing*, *31*(3), 200–207. https://doi.org/10.1016/j.profnurs.2014.11.002

Ronka, S., Karjalainen, K., Martikainen, P., & Makela, P. (2017). Social determinants of drug-related mortality in a general population. *Drug and Alcohol Dependence*, *181*, 37–43. https://doi.org/10.1016/j.drugalcdep.2017.09.005

Roy-Byrne, P., Bumgardner, K., Krupski, A., Dunn, C., Ries, R., Donovan, D., West, I. I., Maynard, C., Atkins, D. C., Graves, M. C., Joesch, J. M., & Zarkin, G. A. (2014). Brief intervention for problem drug users in safety-net primary care settings: A randomized control trial. *Journal of the American Medical Association*, *312*(5), 492–501. https://doi.org/10.1001/jama.2014.7860

Rubinsky, A. D., Kivlahan, D. R., Volk, R. J., Maynard, C., & Bradley, K. A. (2010). Estimating risk of alcohol dependence using alcohol screening scores. *Drug and Alcohol Dependence*, *108*(1–2), 29–36. https://doi.org/10.1016/j.drugalcdep.2009. 11.009

Saitz, R. (2007). Screening and brief intervention enter their 5th decade. *Substance Abuse*, *28*(3), 3–6. https://doi.org/10.1300/J465v28n03_02.

Saitz, R, Palfai, T. A., Cheng, D. M., Alford, D. P., Bernstein, J. A., Lloyd-Travaglini, C. A., Meli, S. M., Chaisson, C. E., & Samet, J. H. (2014). Screening and brief intervention for drug use in primary care: The ASPIRE randomized clinical trial. *Journal of the American Medical Association*, *312*(5), 502–513. https://doi.org/10. 1001/jama.2014.7862

Saunders, J. B., Aasland, O. G., Babor, T. F., de la Fuente, J. R., & Grant, M. (1993). Development of the alcohol use disorders identification test (AUDIT): WHO collaborative project on early detection of persons with harmful alcohol consumption-II. *Addiction*, *88*(6), 791-804. https://doi.org/10.1111/j.1360-0443.1993.tb02093.x

Savage, C., Dyehouse, J., & Marcus, M. (2014). Alcohol and health content in nursing baccalaureate degree curricula. *Journal of Addictions Nursing, 25*(1), 28–34. https://doi.org/10.1097/JAN.0000000000000018

Sawyer, W., & Wagner, P. (2019, March 19). Mass incarceration: The whole pie 2019. *Prison Policy Initiative.* https://www.prisonpolicy.org/reports/pie2019.html

Schieferle Uhlenbrock, J., Fornili, K., & Strobbe, S. (in press). Expanding roles and responsibilities for nurses in screening, brief intervention, and referral to treatment (SBIRT) for alcohol and other substance use: A joint position statement from the Emergency Nurses Association and the International Nurses Society on Addictions. *Journal of Addictions Nursing.*

Schillie, S., Wester, C., Osborne, M., Wesolowski, L., & Ryerson, A. B. (2020, April 10). CDC recommendations for hepatitis c screening among adults—United States, 2020. *MMWR Recommendations and Reports, 69*(2), 1–17. http://dx.doi.org/10.15585/mmwr.rr6902a1

Schmidt, L., Jacobs, L., Vlahov, D., Spetz, J. (2019, Jan 04). Impacts of medical marijuana laws on young Americans across the developmental spectrum. *Journal of Maternal Child & Health, 23*(4), 486–495. https://doi.org/10.1007/s10995-018-2656-1

Scholl, L., Seth, P., Kariisa, M., Wilson, N., Baldwin, G. (2019). Drug and opioid-involved overdose deaths—United States, 2013–2017. *Morbidity and Mortality Weekly Report, 67*(5152), 1419–1427. http://dx.doi.org/10.15585/mmwr.mm675152e1

Semlyen, J., King, M., Varney, J., & Hargar-Johnson, G. (2016). Sexual orientation and symptoms of common mental disorder or low wellbeing: Combined meta-analysis of 12 UK population health surveys. *BMC Psychiatry, 16*(1), 67. https://doi.org/10.1186/s12888-016-0767-z

Smiley, R., Lauer, P., Bienemy, C., Berg, J., Shireman, E., Reneeu, K., & Alexander, M. (2019, January). The 2017 National Nursing Workforce Survey. *Journal of Nursing Regulation, 9*(3, Suppl.), S1–S88. https://doi.org/10.1016/S2155-8256(18)30131-5

Smit, K., Voogt, C., Otten, R., Kleinjan, M., & Kuntsche, E. (2020). Alcohol expectations change in early to middle adolescence as a function of exposure to parental alcohol use. *Drug and Alcohol Dependence, 211*, 107938. https://doi.org/10.1016/j.drugalcdep.2020.107938

Smith, P. C., Cheng, D. M., Allensworth-Davies, D., Winter, M. R., & Saitz, R. (2014). Use of a single alcohol screening question to identify other drug use. *Drug and Alcohol Dependence, 139*, 178–180. https://doi.org/10.1016/j.drugalcdep.2014.03.027

Smith, P. C., Schmidt, S. M., Allensworth-Davies, D., & Saitz, R. (2010). A single-question screening test for drug use in primary care. *Archives of Internal Medicine, 170*(13), 1155–1160. https://doi.org/10.1001/archinternmed.2010.140

Strobbe, S., & Crowley, M. (2017). Substance use among nurses and nursing students: A joint position statement of the Emergency Nurses Association and the International Nurses Society on Addictions. *Journal of Addictions Nursing, 28*(2), 104–106. https://doi.org/10.1097/JAN.0000000000000150

Substance Abuse and Mental Health Services Administration. (n.d.-a). *Evidence-based practices resource center*. https://www.samhsa.gov/ebp-resource-center

Substance Abuse and Mental Health Services Administration. (n.d.-b) *Disclosure of substance use disorder patient records: Does Part 2 apply to me?* https://www.samhsa.gov/sites/default/files/does-part2-apply.pdf

Substance Abuse and Mental Health Services Administration. (2012a). *SAMHSA's working definition of recovery: 10 guiding principles of recovery*. https://store.samhsa.gov/sites/default/files/d7/priv/pep12-recdef.pdf

Substance Abuse and Mental Health Services Administration. (2012b). *Top health issues for LGBT populations: Information & resource kit* (HHS Publication No. [SMA] 12-4684). https://store.samhsa.gov/sites/default/files/d7/priv/sma12-4684.pdf

Substance Abuse and Mental Health Services Administration. (2012c, January). *TIP 54: Managing chronic pain in adults with or in recovery from substance use disorders* (HHS Publication No. [SMA] 13-4671). https://store.samhsa.gov/product/TIP-54-Managing-Chronic-Pain-in-Adults-With-or-in-Recovery-From-Substance-Use-Disorders/SMA13-4671

Substance Abuse and Mental Health Services Administration. (2012d, August). *A Provider's introduction to substance abuse treatment for lesbian, gay, bisexual, and transgender individuals* (HHS Publication No. [SMA] 12–4104). https://store.samhsa.gov/product/A-Provider-s-Introduction-to-Substance-Abuse-Treatment-for-Lesbian-Gay-Bisexual-and-Transgender-Individuals/SMA12-4104

Substance Abuse and Mental Health Services Administration. (2013, May). *TAP 33: Systems-level implementation of screening, brief intervention, and referral to treatment* (HHS Publication No. [SMA] 13-4741). https://store.samhsa.gov/product/TAP-33-Systems-Level-Implementation-of-Screening-Brief-Intervention-and-Referral-to-Treatment-SBIRT/SMA13-4741

Substance Abuse and Mental Health Services Administration. (2014a). *TIP 59: Improving cultural competence* (HHS Publication No. [SMA] 15-4849). https://store.samhsa.gov/product/TIP-59-Improving-Cultural-Competence/SMA15-4849

Substance Abuse and Mental Health Services Administration. (2014b). *TIP 57: Trauma-informed care in behavioral health services* (HHS Publication No. [SMA] 14-4801). https://store.samhsa.gov/product/TIP-57-Trauma-Informed-Care-in-Behavioral-Health-Services/SMA14-4816

Substance Abuse and Mental Health Services Administration. (2014c, February). *A practitioner's resource guide: Helping families to support their LGBT children*. https://store.samhsa.gov/system/files/pep14-lgbtkids.pdf

Substance Abuse and Mental Health Services Administration. (2014d, July). *SAMHSA's concept of trauma and guidance for a trauma-informed approach* (HHS Publication No. [SMA] 14-4884). https://ncsacw.samhsa.gov/userfiles/files/SAMHSA_Trauma.pdf

Substance Abuse and Mental Health Services Administration. (2018, September). *Key substance use and mental health indicators in the United States: Results from the*

2017 National Survey on Drug Use and Health (HHS Publication No. SMA18-5068, NSDUH Series H-53). https://www.samhsa.gov/data/sites/default/files/cbhsq-reports/NSDUHFFR2017/NSDUHFFR2017.pdf

Substance Abuse and Mental Health Services Administration. (2019a, June). *A guide to SAMHSA's strategic prevention framework.* https://www.samhsa.gov/sites/default/files/20190620-samhsa-strategic-prevention-framework-guide.pdf

Substance Abuse and Mental Health Services Administration. (2019b, October). *TIP 35: Enhancing motivation for change in substance use disorder treatment* (SAMHSA Publication No. PEP19-02-01-003). https://store.samhsa.gov/product/TIP-35-Enhancing-Motivation-for-Change-in-Substance-Use-Disorder-Treatment/PEP19-02-01-003

Substance Abuse and Mental Health Services Administration. (2020a, March). *TIP 42: Substance use disorder treatment for people with co-occurring disorders* (SAMHSA Publication No. PEP20-02-01-004). https://store.samhsa.gov/product/tip-42-substance-use-treatment-persons-co-occurring-disorders/PEP20-02-01-004

Substance Abuse and Mental Health Services Administration. (2020b, March 19). *Opioid Treatment Program (OTP) guidance.* https://www.samhsa.gov/sites/default/files/otp-guidance-20200316.pdf

Substance Abuse and Mental Health Services Administration. (2020c, April 23). *Prevention of substance use and mental disorders.* https://www.samhsa.gov/find-help/prevention

Substance Abuse and Mental Health Services Administration. (2020d, April 23). *Recovery and recovery support.* https://www.samhsa.gov/find-help/recovery

Substance Abuse and Mental Health Services Administration. (2020e, May). *TIP 63: Medications for opioid use disorder* (SAMHSA Publication No. PEP20-02-01-006). https://store.samhsa.gov/product/TIP-63-Medications-for-Opioid-Use-Disorder-Full-Document/PEP21-02-01-002

Substance Abuse and Mental Health Services Administration. (2020f, August 19). *MAT medications, counseling, and related conditions.* https://www.samhsa.gov/medication-assisted-treatment/medications-counseling-related-conditions

Substance Abuse and Mental Health Services Administration. (2022a, January 3). *Become a buprenorphine waivered practitioner.* https://www.samhsa.gov/medication-assisted-treatment/become-buprenorphine-waivered-practitioner

Substance Abuse and Mental Health Services Administration. (2022b, January 24). *Buprenorphine.* https://www.samhsa.gov/medication-assisted-treatment/medications-counseling-related-conditions/buprenorphine

Sukel, K. (2019, August 1). *Neurotransmitters.* Dana Foundation. https://www.dana.org/article/neurotransmitters/

Szalavitz, M. (2016, May 10). Opioid addiction is a huge problem, but pain prescriptions are not the cause. *Scientific American.* https://blogs.scientificamerican.com/

mind-guest-blog/opioid-addiction-is-a-huge-problem-but-pain-prescriptions-are-not-the-cause/

Tam, J., Warner, K. E., Meza, M. (2016). Smoking and the reduced life expectancy of individuals with serious mental illness. *American Journal of Prevention Medicine, 51*(6), 958–966. https://doi.org/10.1016/j.amepre.2016.06.007

Thielking, M. (2017, December 21). Life expectancy in the U.S. is falling—and drug overdose deaths are soaring. *Scientific American.* https://www.scientificamerican.com/article/life-expectancy-in-the-u-s-is-falling-and-drug-overdose-deaths-are-soaring/

Thomas, A. A. (2020). Co-occurring pain and addiction. In A. J. Herron & T. K. Brennan (Eds.). *The ASAM essentials of addiction medicine* (3rd ed., pp. 573–577). Wolters Kluwer.

Toledo, L. A. (2017, June 23). Medicaid is the single largest source of care for Americans with mental health, substance use disorders. *The Pulse.* http://pulse.ncpolicywatch.org/2017/06/23/medicaid-single-largest-source-care-americans-mental-health-substance-abuse-disorders/

United Nations Office on Drugs and Crime. (2013). *International standards on drug use prevention.* https://www.unodc.org/documents/prevention/UNODC_2013_2015_international_standards_on_drug_use_prevention_E.pdf

U.S. Department of Health and Human Services. (2016, November). *Office of the Surgeon General, facing addiction in America: The Surgeon General's Report on alcohol, drugs, and health.* https://addiction.surgeongeneral.gov/sites/default/files/surgeon-generals-report.pdf

U.S. Department of Justice Drug Enforcement Agency. (n.d.) *Drug scheduling.* https://www.dea.gov/drug-information/drug-scheduling

U.S. Department of Justice Drug Enforcement Agency. (2020, March 31). *Letter to DEA qualifying practitioners.* https://www.deadiversion.usdoj.gov/GDP/(DEA-DC-022)(DEA068)%20DEA%20SAMHSA%20buprenorphine%20telemedicine%20%20(Final)%20+Esign.pdf

U.S. Food & Drug Administration. (2021, December 17). *Risk evaluation and mitigation strategies: REMS.* https://www.fda.gov/drugs/drug-safety-and-availability/risk-evaluation-and-mitigation-strategies-rems

Vestal, C. (2017, February 6). ACA repeal seen thwarting state addiction efforts. *Stateline Daily.* https://www.pewtrusts.org/en/research-and-analysis/blogs/stateline/2017/02/06/aca-repeal-seen-thwarting-state-addiction-efforts

Volkow, N. D. (2020, April 2). Collision of the COVID-19 and addiction epidemics. *Annals of Internal Medicine.* https://doi.org/10.7326/M20-1212

Volkow, N. D., Baler, R., Compton, W., & Weiss, S. (2014). Adverse health effects of marijuana use. *New England Journal of Medicine, 370*(23), 2219–2227. https://doi.org/10.1056/NEJMra1402309

Volkow, N. D., Swanson, J. M., Evins, A. E., DeLisi, L. E., Meier, M. H., Gonzales, R., Bloomfield, M. A. P., Curran, H. V., & Baler, R. (2016). Effects of cannabis use on human behavior, including cognition, motivation, and psychosis: A review. *JAMA Psychiatry, 73*(3), 714–716. https://doi.org/10.1001/jamapsychiatry.2015.3278

Voss, W. D., Kaufman, E., O'Connor, S. S., Comtois, K. A., Conner, K. R., & Ries, R. K. (2013). Preventing addiction related suicide: A pilot study. *Journal of Substance Abuse Treatment, 44*(5), 565–569. https://doi.org/10.1016/j.jsat.2012.10.006

Vourakis, C. (1996). Addictions nursing practice is knowledge-specific. *Journal of Addictions Nursing, 8*(1), 2–3. https://doi.org/10.3109/10884609609022189

Vourakis, C., and Bennett, G. (1979). Angel dust: Not heaven sent. *American Journal of Nursing, 79*(4), 649–653. https://doi.org/10.2307/3462335

Ward, B., Dahlhamer, J., Galinsky, A., & Joestl, S. (2014). Sexual orientation and health among U.S. adults: National Health Interview Survey, 2013. *National Health Statistics Reports,* (77), 1–10.

Weiss, A., Heslin, K., Barrett, M., Izar, R., & Bierman, A. (2018, September). *Opioid-related inpatient stays and emergency department visits among patients aged 65 years and older, 2010 and 2015* (Statistical brief #244). Agency for Healthcare Research and Quality. https://www.hcup-us.ahrq.gov/reports/statbriefs/sb244-Opioid-Inpatient-Stays-ED-Visits-Older-Adults.jsp

White, W. L. (2008, August). *Recovery management and recovery-oriented systems of care: Scientific rationale and promising practices.* Northeast Addiction Technology Transfer Center, the Great Lakes Addiction Technology Transfer Center, and the Philadelphia Department of Behavioral Health/Mental Retardation Services. http://williamwhitepapers.com/pr/2008RecoveryManagementMonograph.pdf

Wilcox, H. C., Conner, K. R., & Caine, E. D. (2004). Association of alcohol and drug use disorders and completed suicide: An empirical review of cohort studies. *Drug and Alcohol Dependence, 76*(Suppl.), S11–S19. https://doi.org/10.1016/j.drugalcdep.2004.08.003

Wildeman, C., & Wang, E. A. (2017). Mass incarceration, public health, and widening inequality in the USA. *Lancet, 389*(10077), 1464–1474. https://doi.org/10.1016/S0140-6736(17)30259-3

Winkelman, T. N., Chang, V. W., & Binswanger, I. A. (2018). Health, polysubstance use, and criminal justice involvement among adults with varying levels of opioid use. *JAMA Network Open, 1*(3), e180558. https://doi.org/10.1001/jamanetworkopen.2018.0558

Wolf, M., & Rock, L. (2020). EVALI: New information on vaping induced lung injury. *Harvard Health Publishing.* https://www.health.harvard.edu/blog/evali-new-information-on-vaping-induced-lung-injury-2020040319359

Wood, T., Bordelon, C., & Fogger, S. (2019). Shining a light: Integrating protocols into clinical practice for treatment of neonatal abstinence syndrome. *Journal of Addictions Nursing, 30*(1), 61–66. https://doi.org/10.1097/JAN.0000000000000267

World Health Organization. (2018, September 27). *The global status report on alcohol and health 2018.* https://www.who.int/publications/i/item/global-status-report-on-alcohol-and-health-2018

Wright, T., Cluver, J., & Myrick, H. (2020). Management of intoxication and withdrawal: General principles. In A. J. Herron & T. K. Brennan (Eds.), *The ASAM essentials of addiction medicine* (3rd ed., pp. 285–289). Wolters Kluwer.

Yau, Y., Yip, S., & Potenza, M. (2020). Understanding "behavioral addiction." In A. Herron & T. Brennan (Eds.) *The ASAM essentials of addiction medicine* (3rd ed., pp. 250–254). American Society of Addiction Medicine.

Zajicek, A., & Karan, L. (2020). Pharmacokinetic, pharmacodynamic, and pharmacogenomic principles. In A. J. Herron & T. K. Brennan (Eds.), *The ASAM essentials of addiction medicine* (3rd ed., pp. 40–43). Wolters Kluwer.

Zur, J., & Henry, J. (2017). *6 things to know about uninsured adults with opioid addiction* [Fact sheet]. Henry J. Kaiser Family Foundation. https://files.kff.org/attachment/Fact-Sheet-6-Things-to-Know-About-Uninsured-Adults-with-Opioid-Addiction

Appendix A: Addictions Nursing Practice Analysis and Role Delineation Study (2017–2018)

To ensure that the Certified Addictions Registered Nurse (CARN) and Certified Addictions Registered Nurse-Advanced Practice (CARN-AP) certification exams reflect current practice and are legally defensible and psychometrically sound, a 2017–2018 Practice Analysis/Role Delineation survey was conducted by the Center for Nursing Education and Testing (CNET; Garbin, 2019a, 2019b). The study was conducted to describe the activities of specialty nurses (e.g., CARNs and CARN-APs) in enough detail to provide a basis to inform future activities related to certification, including certification examinations. This is a dynamic process that is reevaluated at regular intervals, as required by the Accreditation Board for Specialty Nursing Practice (ABSNC).

The survey collected information from two subgroups of addictions nurses about patient care and work activities, then asked them to rate the frequency and importance of those. The registered nurse (RN) survey (for whom the CARN examination is designed) was completed by nurses prepared at the RN level or those with a graduate degree in areas other than nursing and working in roles other than advanced nursing practice. The advanced practice registered nurse (APRN) survey (for whom the CARN-AP examination is designed) was completed by those prepared for advanced practice (master's degree or higher) and working in the advanced practice nursing role.

REGISTERED NURSE SURVEY RESULTS

The RN survey sample included respondents from 30 states in the United States and Canada. The majority of the RN group was female (89.1%) and White (89.1%). The largest proportion of the RN sample reported their highest degree in nursing was a bachelor's degree (47.5%), followed by associate degree (24.8%), master's (16.1%), and diploma in nursing (8%). RNs responding to the survey had worked as an RN for an average of 22.8 years, with 13.3 years in the addictions nursing specialty and 7.9 years in their current position (Garbin, 2019b).

Among RNs surveyed, the majority (34.4%) worked in outpatient treatment centers, followed by inpatient acute care (25%), inpatient residential treatment centers (23.4%), hospital units (21.9%), mental health facilities/clinics (14.6%), and outreach/community health center settings (8%). Academia, private practice, telehealth, or military was chosen by fewer than 7%. Home health care and school-based clinics accounted for less than 4% (Garbin, 2019b).

The vast majority of respondents (83.9%) reported that they provide direct patient care. The greatest proportion of the RNs (46.9%) reported roles as a clinical nurse, consultant, or provider of other direct patient care services, with an additional 13.7% in case management.

When asked about the percentage of time spent in performing their various duties, about half of their time (53.1%) was spent in providing direct patient care, followed by 20.2% spent in administration (management, supervision, or clerical duties) and 16.5% spent in consultation with providers/care coordination. The nurses spent 6.4% of their time in community outreach/education and 2% in telehealth, marketing, or other activities. Almost all of the respondents (92%–94%) reported working with patients between the ages of 22 and 60 years of age.

ADVANCE PRACTICE REGISTERED NURSE SURVEY RESULTS

The APRN survey included 108 respondents from 35 states in the United States and Canada (Garbin, 2019a). The majority of the APRN respondents were female (88.9%) and White (87%). The largest proportion of the APRN sample reported their highest degree in nursing was a master's (47.2%), followed by a doctorate (30.6%), then a post-master's certificate (13%). The majority of those with doctorates in nursing were DNPs (69.7%) followed by PhDs (15.2%). Of respondents with a non-nursing doctorate (9.3%), most were PhDs and EdDs.

Among the APRN survey respondents, nearly three quarters were nationally certified as nurse practitioners (NP only = 55.6%; both NP and clinical nurse specialist [CNS] = 17.6%), and 17.6% were CNS only. The APRNs reported that they had worked as an RN for an average of 29 years and more than 9 years as an APRN, with more than 13 years in the addictions nursing specialty. On average, APRNs had worked 7 years in their current position (Garbin, 2019a).

The surveyed APRNs practiced in multiple settings. The majority practiced in outpatient treatment centers (44.4%), followed by "other settings" (21.3%). The latter included acute care (emergency department or inpatient care: 17.6%), psychiatric facilities (15.7%), residential treatment centers (13%), community mental health settings (12%), public health/community health centers (9.3%), colleges or universities (7.4%), or methadone clinics (6.5%). Student health and a correctional facility were selected by one respondent each (Garbin, 2019a).

The APRNs spent the most time in direct patient care (58.7%), followed by education of patients, staff, and students (13.2%); care coordination (6.8%); and consultation (6.1%). They also reported spending 4.2% of time in clinical supervision (peer review, precepting, mentoring) and 3% in remaining activities (e.g., research, quality management).

The majority of the APRN respondents worked as a nurse practitioner (66.7%), followed by CNS (16.7%), faculty (7.4%), and managers or administrators (3.7%). Other reported roles included research or owner of practice. The majority of APRNs (81.5%) reported having prescriptive authority, and a third (33.3%) of nurse practitioners had hospital privileges, with more serving in consultation or rounding/follow-up than admitting or discharge.

CONCLUSIONS FOR THE PRACTICE ANALYSIS AND ROLE DELINEATION STUDIES

The Addictions Nursing Practice Analysis and Role Delineation studies describe activities pertaining to the addictions nursing role to ensure that the CARN and the CARN-AP examinations reflect current clinical practice. Complete reports for the most recent CARN and CARN-AP studies can be found on the Addictions Nursing Certification Board (ANCB) website at https://ancbonline.org/Statistics-&-Studies.

The CARN and the CARN-AP practice analysis task forces, with the assistance of C-NET, have evaluated the results of each survey and assigned proposed weights for the distribution of future certification exam content (the "exam blueprints"). The blueprints are available in the Candidate Handbook/Application for the CARN and the CARN-AP found at www.cnetnurse.com.

Glossary

42 CFR Part 2 regulations: Federal regulations that restrict the disclosure and use of "patient-identifying" information about individuals in treatment for substance use, for example, whether a person is receiving, has received, or has applied for treatment for substance use (42 CFR § 2.11). Generally, 42 CFR Part 2 imposes more strict standards than the HIPAA Privacy Rule. 42 CFR Part 2 regulations apply to holders, recipients, and seekers of patient-identifying information. An individual or program in possession of such information may not release or rerelease it except as authorized by the patient concerned or as otherwise permitted by the regulations (42 CFR § 2.13-b). Note: Substance use disorder providers are subject to both 42 CFR Part 2 and the HIPAA Privacy Rule. When one regulation imposes a stricter standard than the other, the provider must follow the stricter standard.

Abstinence: Not using alcohol or drugs (U.S. DHHS, 2016).

Abstinence-based approach: *See also Harm reduction.* An abstinence-based approach is one that requires that patients completely abstain from all substance use and compulsive behaviors. This treatment philosophy is based on beliefs that individuals with addictive disorders cannot use substances or engage in their problematic behaviors in moderation, without loss of control, compulsivity, and related negative consequences.

Abuse: *See Substance abuse.*

Abuse liability: The likelihood that a medication with central nervous system activity will cause desirable psychological effects, such as euphoria or mood changes, that promote misuse of the medication (SAMHSA, 2020e).

Addiction: *See also Physical dependence and Psychological dependence.* A complex condition in which the individual has continued engagement in a behavior despite adverse consequences, diminished self-control over engagement in the behavior, compulsive engagement in the behavior, and an urge or craving state prior to engagement in the behavior (Yau et al., 2020). Addiction has been commonly associated with the use of substances, but the term has more recently been used to describe excessive engagement in problematic nondrug behaviors ("behavioral" or "process" addictions such as eating or sexual disorders and problematic internet use or gambling). Like other chronic illnesses, addiction often involves cycles of relapse and remission. The *Diagnostic and Statistical Manual of Mental Disorders*, fifth edition (*DSM-5*), published by the American Psychiatric Association (APA, 2013) does not use the term "addiction" for diagnostic purposes, but it commonly describes the more severe form of substance use disorders (SAMHSA, 2020e).

Addictions nursing: A distinct nursing specialty practice that incorporates nursing science and the therapeutic use of self with knowledge about substance use and addictive disorders. An addictions nurse is a "nurse" as defined in this volume who also has the expertise to provide care across the continuum of addictive disorders, by focusing their efforts on preventing substance use or problematic behaviors, intervening with those who already have risks for developing an addictive disorder, and providing treatment and recovery support services when indicated. Addictions nurses provide care for individuals with substance use, as well as those with other compulsive and harmful behaviors (e.g., "process addictions" like eating or sexual disorders and problematic internet use or gambling).

Agonist: A chemical substance that binds to and activates certain receptors on cells, causing a biological response. Fentanyl and methadone are examples of opioid receptor agonists (U.S. DHHS, 2016).

Ambivalence: A normal part of any change process, perceived as uncomfortable because it involves conflicting motivations about making changes (Miller & Rollnick, 2013).

Antagonist: A chemical substance that binds to and blocks the activation of certain receptors on cells, preventing a biological response. Naloxone is an example of an opioid receptor antagonist (U.S. DHHS, 2016).

At-risk alcohol use: *See also Binge drinking and Heavy drinking*. A term for (1) any drinking by those who are pregnant, underage, operating machinery, or with a health condition adversely affected by alcohol; (2) binge drinking; or (3) heavy drinking. Note: At-risk alcohol use can jeopardize health and safety and increase an individual's risk of developing an alcohol use disorder (AUD), although at-risk alcohol use may not meet diagnostic criteria for AUD (Institute for Research, Education & Training in Addictions, n.d.).

Behavioral addictions: *See Addiction.*

Behavioral health services: The collective term for mental health and substance use disorder services; may be considered less stigmatizing than the use of either term alone.

Binge (binge drinking): Pattern of drinking that brings blood alcohol concentration (BAC) levels to 0.08 grams per deciliter (g/dL), which typically occurs after four drinks for women and five drinks for men in about 2 hours (National Institute on Alcohol Abuse and Alcoholism, n.d.).

Brief intervention (BI): *See also Screening and Screening, Brief Intervention, and Referral to Treatment (SBIRT).* BIs are short, motivational interventions appropriate for patients identified through screening to be at risk for substance use problems (Babor & Higgins-Biddle, 2001). BIs can consist of one or more encounters, typically provided at the same site as the screening. The goals of BI are to increase an individual's insight and awareness about their substance use risks and consequences, and the need for behavioral change, based on their level of readiness. Those with mild risks can benefit from a BI, and those with moderate-to-severe risks (or probable substance use disorders) can benefit from multiple BI, or a BI designed to facilitate a referral for a comprehensive biopsychosocial assessment and treatment if indicated.

Buprenorphine: A medication to treat opioid use disorder (MOUD). Buprenorphine is the first MOUD approved by the Food and Drug Administration (FDA) for the treatment of opioid use disorder (OUD) that can be prescribed or dispensed in medical offices, which can significantly increase access to treatment.

Buprenorphine waiver: *See Waiver.*

Compulsivity: Repetitive behaviors in the face of adverse consequences, as well as repetitive behaviors that are inappropriate to a particular situation. People suffering from compulsions often recognize that the behaviors are harmful, but they nonetheless feel emotionally compelled to perform them. Doing so reduces tension, stress, or anxiety (U.S. DHHS, 2016).

Continuum of care: An integrated system of care that guides and tracks a person over time through a comprehensive array of health services appropriate to the individual's need. A continuum of care may include prevention, early intervention, treatment, continuing care, and recovery support (U.S. DHHS, 2016).

Controlled substance: A drug or other substance, or immediate precursor, included in schedule I, II, III, IV, or V of part B of Title 21 United States Code (USC) Controlled Substances Act. The term "controlled substances" does not include distilled spirits, wine, malt beverages, or tobacco, as those terms are defined or used in subtitle E of the Internal Revenue Code of 1986.

Controlled Substances Act (CSA): Federal law that regulates certain substances by placing them into one of five "schedules," based on their medical use, potential for misuse, and safety or dependence liability. More information can be found in Title 21 United States Code (USC) Controlled Substances Act.

Co-occurring disorders: Any combination of two disorders or illnesses coexisting at the same time. Although co-occurring disorders can refer to any two diagnoses, it most commonly refers to the coexistence of both a substance use disorder and a psychiatric illness.

Cross-tolerance: *See also Tolerance and Sensitization.* Cross-tolerance is a change in the way that the body responds that occurs when tolerance to repeated use of a specific drug in a given category is generalized to other drugs in the same structural and mechanistic category. For example, the cross-tolerance that occurs between alcohol, barbiturates, and benzodiazepines can be used to facilitate the smooth weaning of a patient from their drug of choice during detoxification (Zajicek & Karan, 2020).

Dependence: *See Substance dependence.*

Detoxification: *See also Medically supervised withdrawal and Withdrawal management.* Detoxification usually refers to a process of withdrawing a person from a specific psychoactive substance in a safe and effective manner. The term has been replaced by the terms "medically supervised withdrawal" or "withdrawal management" (Mee-Lee et al., 2013, p. 418).

Diagnostic and Statistical Manual of Mental Disorders (DSM): The taxonomic and diagnostic tool published by the American Psychiatric Association (APA). Addictions nurses in the United States refer to the diagnostic criteria and terminology in this publication to inform their practice.

Dissociation: Rate at which a drug uncouples from a receptor. A drug with a longer dissociation rate will have a longer duration of action than a drug with a shorter dissociation rate (SAMHSA, 2020e).

Diversion (drug diversion): A medical and legal concept involving the transfer of any legally prescribed controlled substance from the person for whom it was prescribed to another person for any illicit use (U.S. DHHS, 2016).

Early intervention: Services for early recognition of a problem (screening) and minimization of harm (Babor et al., 1986), especially among individuals who have not yet developed the need for extensive, specialized treatment (SAMHSA, 2013).

Euphoria: "A mental and emotional condition in which a person experiences intense feelings of well-being, elation, happiness, excitement, and joy" (APA, 2013, p. 821).

Gender: "The public (and usually legally recognized) lived role as a boy or girl, man or woman. Biological factors are seen as contributing interactionally with social and psychological factors to gender development" (APA, 2013, p. 822).

Gender identity: A personal sense of having a particular gender, which may develop in early life. Gender identity refers to how people feel about their gender on the inside and how they express their gender through clothing choices, behaviors, and personal appearance.

Half-life: Rate of removal of a drug from the body. One half-life removes 50% of the drug from the plasma. After a drug is stopped, it takes five half-lives to remove about 95% of the drug from the body. If a drug is continued at the same dose, its plasma level will continue to rise until it reaches steady state concentrations after about five half-lives (SAMHSA, 2020e).

Harm reduction: *See also Abstinence-based approach.* Harm reduction refers to person-centered, population health interventions that aim to reduce negative effects of substance use and other risky health behaviors, without necessarily requiring abstinence or completely extinguishing the behavior. Examples include promoting needle exchange programs to reduce needle sharing, encouraging bar patrons to get a cab while drinking to reduce driving under the influence, or offering condoms to promote safer sex.

Health disparities: Preventable differences in the burden of disease or opportunities to achieve optimal health that are experienced by socially disadvantaged populations, defined by factors such as race or ethnicity, gender, education or income, disability, geographic location (e.g., rural or urban), and sexual orientation (U.S. DHHS, 2016).

Heavy drinking: Defined by the Centers for Disease Control and Prevention (CDC) as consuming 8 or more drinks per week for women and 15 or more drinks per week for men, and by the Substance Abuse and Mental Health Services Administration (SAMHSA), for research purposes, as binge drinking on 5 or more days in the past 30 days (U.S. DHHS, 2016).

Impulsivity: Inability to resist urges, deficits in delaying gratification, and unreflective decision-making. Impulsivity is a tendency to act without foresight or regard for consequences and to prioritize immediate rewards over long-term goals (U.S. DHHS, 2016).

Induction: Process of initial dosing with medication for opioid use disorder (OUD) treatment until the patient reaches a state of stability; also called initiation (SAMHSA, 2020e).

Intervention: A professionally delivered program, service, or policy designed to prevent substance misuse (prevention intervention) or treat a substance use disorder (treatment intervention; U.S. DHHS, 2016).

Intoxication: "The result of being under the influence of, and responding to, the acute effects of alcohol or another drug. Intoxication states can range from euphoria or sedation to life-threatening emergencies when overdose occurs. Each substance has a set of signs and symptoms that are seen during intoxication" (Wright et al., 2020, p. 285).

LGBTQIA: Acronym for lesbian, gay, bisexual, transgender, queer, intersex, and asexual (specific definitions for each of these terms are in the LGBTQIA section of the *Scope and Standards* under Special Populations).

Maintenance treatment: Providing medications to achieve and sustain clinical remission of the signs and symptoms of substance use disorders (SUD) and to support the individual process of recovery without a specific endpoint, as per the typical standard of care for other chronic illnesses (SAMHSA, 2020e).

Medically supervised withdrawal: *See also Detoxification and Withdrawal management.* Medically supervised withdrawal (formerly called detoxification) refers to the use of a medication in tapering doses to help a patient with dependence discontinue the use of illicit or prescription medications. For example, for patients with opioid dependence, medically supervised withdrawal may involve using an opioid agonist or an alpha-2 adrenergic agonist if opioid agonist is not available (SAMHSA, 2020e).

Medical management: Process whereby nurses and other health care professionals provide medication, basic brief supportive counseling, monitoring of drug use and medication adherence, and when necessary, referrals to addiction counseling and other services to address the patient's medical, mental health, comorbid addiction, and psychosocial needs (SAMHSA, 2020e).

Medication-assisted treatment (MAT): *See also Medications for opioid use disorder (MOUD).* "Medication-assisted treatment" is an outdated, stigmatizing term that has now been replaced by "medications for opioid use disorder" (MOUD) or "medications for addictions treatment" (also MAT). The word "assisted" implies that medications like methadone, buprenorphine, or naltrexone are "partial treatments," not primary treatments for opioid use disorder (OUD), alcohol use disorder (AUD), or other substance use disorders (SUD). The term "assisted" relegates medications for addictions treatment to a less desirable status than medications for other chronic disorders. Some addictions advocates believe that the word "assisted" leads to further stigmatization of people with SUD, in that it implies that they are "not really in recovery" or are "replacing one substance with another." Many people can benefit greatly from counseling or other psychosocial therapies, but these therapies are not always required for pharmacological treatment to be successful, and medications for SUD save lives.

Medications for opioid use disorder (MOUD): *See also Medication-assisted treatment (MAT).* Preferred term for pharmacological treatment of opioid use disorders using medications such as methadone, buprenorphine, and naltrexone; formerly referred to with the outdated term medication-assisted treatment (MAT).

Methadone: A medication to treat opioid use disorder (MOUD), as well as for pain management. When taken as prescribed, methadone is safe and effective. Methadone helps individuals to achieve and sustain recovery and to reclaim active and meaningful lives. A long-acting opioid agonist, methadone reduces opioid craving and withdrawal and blunts or blocks the effects of opioids. By law, only a SAMHSA-certified opioid treatment program (OTP) can dispense methadone for the treatment of OUD.

Misuse: *See Substance misuse*

Morphine milligram equivalents (MME): The milligrams of morphine an opioid dose is equal to when prescribed. Calculating MME accounts for differences in opioid drug types and strengths.

Motivation: A multidimensional, fluid state during which people make difficult changes to health-risk behaviors like substance misuse; a critical element of behavior change that predicts abstinence and reductions in substance use (SAMHSA, 2019b).

Motivational interviewing (MI): Created by William Miller and Stephen Rollnick, MI is the most widely researched and disseminated counseling approach in substance use disorder treatment, brief interventions (BI) for substance misuse in the Screening, Brief Intervention, and Referral to Treatment (SBIRT) model, and other health promotion interventions. It is a philosophical approach to working with patients as much as it is a therapeutic technique, as it incorporates Rodgerian principles of positive regard for the individual in exploring and resolving ambivalence toward change and empowers people to take responsibility for their own recovery.

Mutual-help groups: Groups of people who work together on obtaining and maintaining recovery. Unlike "peer support" (e.g., use of recovery coaches), mutual help groups consist entirely of people who volunteer their time and typically have no official connection to treatment programs. Most are self-supporting. Although twelve-step groups such as Alcoholics Anonymous (AA) and Narcotic Anonymous (NA) are the most widespread and well-researched type of mutual-help groups, other secular and nonsecular groups may be available in some areas (SAMHSA, 2020e).

Naloxone (Narcan): A short-acting opioid antagonist medicine that rapidly reverses an opioid overdose by attaching to opioid receptors and reversing and blocking the effects of other opioids. Naloxone can quickly restore normal breathing to a person if their breathing has slowed or stopped because of an opioid overdose. However, naloxone has no effect on someone who does not have opioids in their system, and it is not a treatment for opioid use disorder. Emergency overdose kits available to the public typically contain the nasal spray form or the auto-inject form of naloxone for first aid treatment of opioid overdose.

Naltrexone: *See also Risk Evaluation and Mitigation Strategy (REMS).* Naltrexone is a medication for addictions treatment (MAT) approved by the Food and Drug Administration (FDA) to treat both opioid use disorder (OUD) and alcohol use disorder (AUD). Naltrexone can be prescribed and administered by any practitioner licensed to prescribe medications and is available in a pill form for AUD or as an extended-release intramuscular injectable for either AUD or OUD. A Risk Evaluation and Mitigation Strategy (REMS) is required for the long-acting injectable formulation to ensure that the benefits of the drug outweigh its risks.

Narcan: *See Naloxone.*

Neurotransmitter: A chemical that acts as a messenger between neurons (nerve cells), and activates numerous biological, psychological, and behavioral processes associated with substance use disorders (Sukel, 2019).

Office-based opioid treatment (OBOT): *See also Opioid treatment programs (OTP).* OBOT refers to the practice of providing medication for the treatment of opioid use disorders in settings other than federally regulated opioid treatment programs—OTPs (SAMHSA, 2020e).

Opiate: Natural opioids such as heroin, morphine, and codeine (CDC, 2021).

Opioid: Natural, synthetic, or semisynthetic chemicals that interact with opioid receptors on nerve cells in the body and brain and reduce the intensity of pain signals and feelings of pain. This class of drugs includes the illegal drug heroin; synthetic opioids, such as fentanyl; and prescribed pain medications, such as oxycodone, hydrocodone, codeine, morphine, and many others (CDC, 2021).

Opioid overdose: *See Overdose.*

Opioid treatment program (OTP): *See also Office-based opioid treatment (OBOT).* An OTP is an accredited treatment program (sometimes referred to as a "methadone clinic") with certification from the U.S. DHHS Substance Abuse and Mental Health Services Administration (SAMHSA) and registration from the U.S. Department of Justice (DOJ) Drug Enforcement Agency (DEA). An OTP may only administer and dispense medications for opioid use disorder that have been approved by the DHHS Food and Drug Administration (FDA) for that indication. At the time of this writing, these medications include methadone and buprenorphine products. Other pharmacotherapies, such as naltrexone, may be provided but are not subject to these regulations. OTPs must provide adequate medical, counseling, vocational, educational, and other services either onsite or by referral to an outside agency or practitioner through a formal agreement (SAMHSA, 2020e).

Overdose: Injury to the body (poisoning) that happens when a drug is taken in excessive amounts. An overdose can be fatal or nonfatal (CDC, 2021). The poisoning can be distinguished by intent: unintentional drug poisoning (accidental overdose), intentional drug poisoning (suicide or attempted suicide), or assault (injuries intended to injure or kill, including homicidal poisoning; Goldberger et al., 2013).

Parity/insurance parity: Federal requirements that health insurance plans cover behavioral health (mental health and substance use) services at the same level as health plans for physical conditions, under the Paul Wellstone and Pete Domenici Mental Health Parity and Addiction Equity Act of 2008 (the *Parity Act*).

Physical dependence: *See also Psychological dependence, Substance dependence, and Withdrawal.* A state of adaptation manifested by a drug class specific withdrawal syndrome produced by abrupt cessation, rapid dose reduction, decreasing blood levels of the drug, and/or administration of an antagonist (Mee-Lee et al., 2013, p. 417). Note: Diminished self-control and compulsive substance use behaviors are the distinguishing features of addiction. Physical dependence does not equate to addiction, and it is not included in the *Diagnostic and Statistical Manual of Mental Disorders*, fifth edition (*DSM-5*) definition of substance use disorder.

Privacy and confidentiality: *See 42 CFR Part 2 regulations.*

Protective factors: Factors that directly decrease the likelihood of substance use and behavioral health problems or reduce the impact of risk factors on behavioral health problems (U.S. DHHS, 2016).

Psychological dependence: *See also Physical dependence, Substance dependence, and Withdrawal.* A subjective sense of need for a specific psychoactive substance, in order to experience the positive effects of the substance or to avoid negative effects when the substance is absent (Mee-Lee et al., 2013, p. 417). Note: As with physical dependence, psychological dependence is not included in the *Diagnostic and Statistical Manual of Mental Disorders*, fifth edition (*DSM-5*) definition of substance use disorder.

Receptor: Molecules on the surfaces of neurons (nerve cells) whose structures precisely match those of chemical messengers (neurotransmitters or hormones). The chemicals attach themselves to the receptors, in lock-and-key fashion, to activate the receiving cell (Sukel, 2019).

Recovery: A process of change through which people improve their health and wellness, live self-directed lives, and strive to reach their full potential. The four major dimensions of wellness that support recovery include health (overcoming or managing one's disease(s) or symptoms and making informed, healthy choices that support physical and emotional well-being), home (having a stable and safe place to live), purpose (conducting meaningful daily activities and having the independence, income, and resources to participate in society), and community (having relationships and social networks that provide support, friendship, love, and hope; SAMHSA, 2020d).

Recovery-oriented care: A service orientation that supports individuals with behavioral health conditions in a process of change through which they can improve their health and wellness, live self-directed lives, and strive to reach their full potential (SAMHSA, 2020e).

Recovery support/Recovery support services (RSS): *See also Wraparound services.* Nonclinical services offered before, during, or in lieu of treatment by nurses and other health professionals as well as family members and peers in recovery. RSS may be provided in a variety of community, faith-based, treatment, or other settings, often over a sustained period. The RSS continuum includes child care, transportation, housing, life skills training, employment readiness, legal consultation, wellness checks, and self-management support (White, 2008).

Relapse: "A process in which an individual who has established abstinence or sobriety experiences recurrence of signs and symptoms of active addiction, often including resumption of the pathological pursuit of reward and/or relief through the use of substances and other behaviors" (Mee-Lee et al., 2013, p. 427). Relapse is different than a return to opioid use in that it involves more than a single incident of use, occurs over a period of time, can be interrupted, and needs not be long lasting (SAMHSA, 2020e).

Relapse prevention: A cognitive-behavioral, self-management program that combines behavioral skill training, cognitive interventions, and lifestyle change procedures; designed to help individuals who are trying to maintain behavioral changes to anticipate and cope with the problem of relapse (Marlatt, 1985).

Risk Evaluation and Mitigation Strategy (REMS): Drug safety program that the U.S. Food and Drug Administration (FDA) can require for certain medications with serious safety concerns to help ensure that the benefits of the medication outweigh its risks. While all medications have labeling that informs health care stakeholders about medication risks, only a few medications require a REMS. The focus of a REMS is on preventing, monitoring, and/or managing a specific serious risk by informing, educating, and/or reinforcing actions to reduce the frequency and/or severity of adverse events (U.S. FDA, 2021).

Risk factors: Factors that increase the likelihood of beginning substance use, of regular and harmful use, and of other behavioral health problems associated with use (U.S. DHHS, 2016).

Screening: *See also Brief intervention (BI).* A process of using a validated instrument to identify individuals with possible substance misuse or a substance use disorder. The screening process is not used for determination of problem severity or for diagnostic purposes. Screening simply determines if the individual *might* have a problem.

Screening, Brief Intervention, and Referral to Treatment (SBIRT): *See also Brief intervention (BI).* An evidence-based, early intervention strategy designed to reduce substance use and related consequences by identifying and intervening with people who have risky alcohol or drug use behaviors before the onset of serious substance-related disorders.

Sensitization: *See also Tolerance.* Tolerance and sensitization reflect the way the body responds to a drug when it is used repeatedly. Sensitization is an increase in response to a drug after repeated administration (Zajicek & Karan, 2020).

Sex: "Biological indication of male and female (understood in the context of reproductive capacity) such as sex chromosomes, gonads, sex hormones, and non-ambiguous internal and external genitalia" (APA, 2013, p. 829).

Social determinants of substance use and addiction: Biological, social, environmental, psychological, and genetic factors associated with substance use and addiction. These factors can include gender, race and ethnicity, age, income level, educational attainment, sexual orientation, and interpersonal, household, and community dynamics.

Standard drink: Based on the 2015–2020 Dietary Guidelines for Americans, a standard drink is defined as 12 fl oz of regular beer, 8–9 fl oz of malt liquor, 5 fl oz of table wine, or 1.5 fl oz of 80-proof distilled spirits. All of these drinks contain 14 grams (0.6 oz) of pure alcohol (U.S. DHHS, 2016).

Stigma: *See also Stigma of addiction.* Negative stereotypes, perceptions, and judgments attributed to a person or groups of people viewed as different or inferior, often based on preconceived, often false ideas and generalizations.

Stigma of addiction: *See also Stigma.* Social prejudices, pejorative attitudes, perceptions, or judgments attributed to persons with substance use or addiction. The stigma of addiction can be a barrier to the development of a therapeutic alliance and the initiation or continuation of an individual's recovery process.

Substance: A psychoactive compound with the potential to cause health and social problems, including substance use disorders and their most severe manifestation, addiction (SAMHSA, 2019b).

Substance abuse: Outdated yet commonly used term for maladaptive pattern of substance use leading to clinically significant impairment or distress. It is now considered to be a stigmatizing term because it is strongly associated with negative judgment and implies that the individual has control over their behaviors or use of substances, chooses to engage in immoral or willful misconduct, and is more deserving of criminal punishment instead of treatment.

Substance dependence: *See also Physical dependence and Psychological dependence.* A state in which an organism only functions normally in the presence of a substance, experiencing physical disturbance when the substance is removed. A person can be dependent on a substance without being addicted, but dependence sometimes leads to addiction (U.S. DHHS, 2016).

Substance misuse: Term used to distinguish use of a prescribed medication or moderate use of alcohol from improper or unhealthy use of those substances. Includes using prescription drugs in ways other than prescribed or using someone else's prescription (National Institute on Drug Abuse, 2018c). It includes the use of any substance in a manner, situation, amount, or frequency that can cause harm to users or to those around them. For some substances or individuals, any use would constitute misuse, for example, underage drinking, injection drug use (SAMHSA, 2019b).

Substance use disorders (SUD): The *Diagnostic and Statistical Manual of Mental Disorders*, fifth edition (*DSM-5*) nomenclature for what previously was referred to as "substance abuse" and "substance dependence" (APA, 2013). SUDs describe significant clinical and functional impairment resulting from the recurrent use of substances; they are defined as mild, moderate, or severe, based on the number of *DSM-5* diagnostic criteria met by an individual.

Tolerance: *See also Sensitization and Cross-tolerance.* Tolerance and sensitization reflect the way the body responds to a drug when it is used repeatedly. Tolerance is the reduction in response to a drug after repeated administration (Zajicek & Karan, 2020).

Treatment: "Application of planned procedures to identify and change patterns of behavior that are maladaptive, destructive, and/or injurious to health; or to restore appropriate levels of physical, psychological, and/or social functioning" (Mee-Lee et al., 2013, p. 432).

Treatment gap: Commonly refers to a phenomenon wherein individuals are classified as needing but not receiving substance use disorder (SUD) treatment.

Treatment of addiction: "The use of any planned, intentional intervention in the health, behavior, personal, and/or family life of an individual suffering from alcohol use disorder or from another drug addiction, and which is designed to facilitate the affected individual to achieve and maintain sobriety, physical, spiritual, and mental health, and a maximum functional ability" (Mee-Lee et al., 2013, p. 432).

Twelve-Step Facilitation: *See also Twelve-step programs and Mutual-help groups.* Semi-structured therapies that utilize active engagement strategies to increase the likelihood of an individual becoming affiliated with, and actively involved in, community-based twelve-step or mutual-help groups.

Twelve-step programs: *See also Mutual help groups and Twelve-Step Facilitation.* A group providing mutual support and fellowship for people recovering from addictive behaviors. The first twelve-step program was Alcoholics Anonymous (AA), founded in 1935; an array of twelve-step groups following a similar model have since emerged and are the most widely used mutual aid groups and steps for maintaining recovery from alcohol and drug use disorders. It is not a form of treatment, and it is not to be confused with the treatment modality called Twelve-Step Facilitation (U.S. Department of Health and Human Services [U.S. DHHS], 2016). Twelve-step programs are based in common spiritual beliefs that a person is powerless over their use of the substance(s) and that a higher power may help them find meaning in their life outside of addiction.

Waiver ("Buprenorphine waiver" or "DATA 2000 waiver" or the "X waiver"): Under the Controlled Substances Act (CSA), practitioners are prohibited from prescribing opioids for the treatment of opioid use disorders (OUD), except for methadone (Schedule II), available only at federally certified opioid treatment programs (OTPs) and acute inpatient hospital settings for OUD treatment (SAMHSA, 2022b). Practitioners may apply for and receive a waiver to prescribe medications that have been approved by the Food and Drug Administration (FDA) for the treatment of OUD outside of OTPs. However, at the time of this writing, buprenorphine products (Schedule III) are the only medications approved by the FDA for that indication. This waiver is commonly referred to as the "buprenorphine waiver", the Drug Addiction Treatment Act of 2000 ("DATA 2000") waiver, or the "X waiver."

Withdrawal: The development of a substance-specific problematic behavioral change, with physiological and cognitive consequences, that is due to cessation of, or reduction in, heavy and prolonged substance use (APA, 2013).

Withdrawal management: *See also Detoxification and Medically supervised withdrawal.*

Wrap-around services: *See also Recovery support/Recovery support services (RSS).* Nonclinical services that facilitate patient engagement and retention in treatment as well as their ongoing recovery. This can include services to address patient needs related to transportation, employment, child care, housing, and legal and financial problems, among others (U.S. DHHS, 2016).

Index

aftercare 92
agencies
    community-based 40
    government 3, 92, 101
    regulatory 105
AGS (American Geriatrics Society) 33
alcohol. *See also* screenings, for alcohol
    problems
    associated rates regarding 29
    binge drinking 29–30
    consumption during pregnancy 27
    heavy use of 31
    older adults use of 33
    underage use of 28–30
    utero exposure to 27–28
Alcoholics Anonymous 59
alcohol use disorder (AUD) 42. *See also* substance use disorders (SUDs)
    medications for 50
Alcohol Use Disorder Identification Test (AUDIT) 42
American Association of Colleges of Nursing (AACN) 18
American Geriatrics Society (AGS) 33
American Medical Society on Alcoholism 9
American Nurses Association (ANA) 1
    organizational affiliates of 14
American Psychiatric Association (APA) 2
American Society of Addiction Medicine (ASAM) 2
    level of care 45–47
Americans with Disabilities Act (ADA) 92
    public accommodations under 93
ANA. *See* American Nurses Association (ANA)
analgesics 80
ANCB (Addictions Nursing Certification Board) 15–16
anticonvulsant drugs 80
antidepressant medications 80
APA (American Psychiatric Association) 2

approaches
    alternative-to-discipline (ATD) 82, 100
    trauma-informed 73
APRNs (advanced practice registered nurses) 21–22
arrests, drug-related 90
ASAM. *See* American Society of Addiction Medicine (ASAM)
asexuality 84
assessment 107–109
    APRN competencies 109
    of competence 97
    competencies 107–109
    comprehensive 41
    graduate-level competencies 109
    multidimensional 44
    of performance 104
    Standard 1 107–109
assurance 105
attention-deficit hyperactivity disorder (ADHD) 77
attitudes 66
    changing of 99
attributes, individual 37
AUD (alcohol use disorder) 42
AUDIT (Alcohol Use Disorder Identification Test) 42
autonomy 58
awareness, addiction 9

B

BAC (blood alcohol concentration) 31
bachelor of science in nursing (BSN) 18
behavioral addictions 3, 62
behavioral health 4
    access to treatment for 88
behavioral therapies 44
behaviors 37, 66
    change processes 96
    compulsive 3
    consequences and 3
    effects of addictive 17
    engagement in 3
    ethical 95
    level of 104

disorders (*continued*)
psychiatric 70, 77
substance use as 96
trauma-related 73
disparities
in arrests 90
in health 84
reduction of 101
Division of Pharmacologic Therapies (DPT) 47
DMV (department of motor vehicles) 93
doctor of nursing practice (DNP) 23
doctor of nursing science degrees (DNS, DSN, or DNSc) 22
DOT (Department of Transportation) 93
DPT (Division of Pharmacologic Therapies) 47
driving under the influence (DUI) 70, 93
Drug Addiction Treatment Act of 2000 (DATA 2000) 89
Drug and Alcohol Nurses Association (DANA) 9
drugs. *See also* controlled substances; medications
anticonvulsant 80
diversion 81
psychoactive use of 17
related arrests 90
testing of 51
DSM-5 (Diagnostic and Statistical Manual of Mental Disorders) 2, 73
DUI (driving under the influence) 70, 93
duties
of nurses 103
to self 98

E

early intervention 40
eating disorders 62, 77
EBPs (evidence-based practices) 23–24
education
baccalaureate-level 18

competencies 129
expertise and 22
gaps in 19
graduate-level 19
services 25
Standard 12 129
EHBs (essential health benefits) 88
EMCDDA (European Monitoring Centre for Drugs and Drug Addiction Best Practices Portal) 36–37
emotional trauma 73
engagement, behavioral 3
Environmental Health (Standard 17) 136–137
APRN competencies 136–137
competencies 136
graduate-level competencies 136–137
environments
ethical 99
factors for 38
health 136–137
promotion of safe 96
equity of health 6
ESNO (European Specialist Nurses Organisation) 15
essential health benefits (EHBs) 88
ethics 121–122
behavioral 95
code of 95
competencies 121–122
concerns in 95
environment and 99
nursing conduct 97
practices 95
Standard 7 121–122
etiologies 3
European Monitoring Centre for Drugs and Drug Addiction Best Practices Portal (EMCDDA) 36–37
European Specialist Nurses Organisation (ESNO) 15
evaluation 39. *See also* Professional Practice Evaluation (Standard 15)

Treatment Improvement Protocol (TIP)
24
twelve-step programs 59

U

United Nations Office on Drugs and
Crime (UNODC) 36
universal human rights 101, 102
UNODC (United Nations Office on
Drugs and Crime) 36
urges 3

V

vaping 29
Volkow, Nora 67
vulnerabilities 36

social 84

W

War on Drugs 90, 91
welfare, child 93
wellness 2
dimensions supporting recovery 4
WHO (World Health Organization) 4
WIA (Workforce Investment Act) 92
withdrawal 96
Workforce Investment Act (WIA) 92
World Health Organization (WHO) 4

Y

Youth Risk Behavior Surveillance
System (YRBSS) 30